Caring for the Rural Community

An Interdisciplinary Curriculum

American
Psychological
Association
Office of
Rural Health

First printing January 1995
Second printing April 1995

Published by
American Psychological Association
750 First Street, NE
Washington, DC 20002

Copies may be ordered from
APA Order Department
P.O. Box 2710
Hyattsville, MD 20784

Typeset in Century by University Graphics, Inc., York, PA

Printer: Wickersham Printing Company, Inc., Lancaster, PA
Technical/Production Editor: Sarah J. Trembath
Cover Designer: Minker Design, Bethesda, MD

Cover photograph by Sunny Reynolds

Library of Congress Cataloging-in-Publication Data

Caring for the rural community : an interdisciplinary curriculum / American Psychological Association, Office of Rural Health.
p. cm.
Includes bibliographical references.
ISBN 1-55798-288-0
1. Rural mental health services—United States. I. American Psychological Association. Office of Rural Health.
[DNLM: 1. Community Mental Health Services—United States. 2. Rural Health—United States. 3. Curriculum. WA 305 C277 1995]
RA790.6.C36 1995
362.2′2′0973—dc20
DNLM/DLC
for Library of Congress 94-49194
CIP

Printed in the United States of America

Contents

Contributors

Planning/Advisory Task Force
Interdisciplinary Team Training Curriculum

Anita Brown, PhD
Assistant Executive Director
APA Practice Directorate
750 First Street, NE
Washington, DC 20002-4242

Ronald D. DePrez, PhD, MPH, *Consultant*
Public Health Resource Group
60 York Street
Portland, ME 04101

Doris Droke, *Project Officer*
Bureau of Health Professions
Room 8C02, Parklawn Building
Fishers Lane
Rockville, MD 20857

E. Aracelis Francis, DSW
Director
Minority Fellowship Programs
Council on Social Work Education
1600 Duke Street
Alexandria, VA 22314-3421

Leon H. Ginsberg, MSW, PhD
Carolina Research Professor
College of Social Work
University of South Carolina
Columbia, SC 29208

Susan M. Godschalx, PhD, RN
Clinical Director
Four Corners Mental Health Center
198 East Center Street
Moab, UT

Gil Hill, *Project Director*
Director, Office of Rural Health
APA Practice Directorate
750 First Street, NE
Washington, DC 20002-4242

Catherine Francis Kane, PhD, RN
Western State Hospital
P.O. Box 2500
Staunton, VA 24402-2500

Peter Keller, PhD
Professor and Chair
Department of Psychology
Mansfield University
Mansfield, PA 16933

Jerry Morris, PsyD
815 South Ash
Nevada, MO 64772

Helen Munoz, MSW
COSSMHO
1501 16th Street, N.W.
Washington, DC 20036

Ralph E. Packard, PhD, *Consultant*
Department of Educational Psychology
327 MBH
University of Utah
Salt Lake City, UT 84112

Wanda Wahnee Priddy, MSW
P.O. Box 1281
Tahlequah, OK 74465

Sarah Stanley, MS, RN
Senior Policy Analyst
American Nurses Association
600 Maryland Avenue, SW
Suite 100 West
Washington, DC 20024-2571

APA Rural Health Task Force

Michael Enright, PhD, *Chair*
P.O. Box 4120
Jackson, WY 83001-4120

Paul Craig, PhD, *Member*
Alaska Guidance and Diagnostic Clinic
Providence Tower Building
3260 Providence Drive, Suite 422
Anchorage, AK 99508-4615

David Scott Hargrove, PhD, *Member*
Professor and Chair
Department of Psychology
University of Mississippi
Oxford, MS 38677

Mary Beth Kenkel, PhD, *Member*
Chancellor
California School of Professional Psychology
1250 M Street
Fresno, CA 93721-1808

James Bray, PhD, *Vice Chair*
Department of Family Medicine
Baylor College of Medicine
5510 Greenbrier
Houston, TX 77005

Arthur McDonald, PhD, *Member*
President
Dull Knife Memorial College
Post Office Box 98
Lame Deer, MT 59043

Jerry Morris, PsyD, *Member*
815 South Ash
Nevada, MO 64772

Sylvia Shellenberger, PhD, *Member*
Family Health Center
3780 Eisenhower Parkway
Macon, GA 31206

Jack G. Wiggins, Jr., PhD, *Senior Advisor*
Psychology Development Center Inc.
7057 West 130th Street
Cleveland, OH 44130

Project Management Committee
Interdisciplinary Team Training Curriculum

Doris Droke, *Project Officer*
Bureau of Health Professions
Room 8C02
Parklawn Building
Fishers Lane
Rockville, MD 20857

Gil Hill, *Project Director*
Director
Marquette W. Turner
Program Assistant
Office of Rural Health
APA Practice Directorate
750 First Street, NE
Washington, DC 20002-4242

E. Aracelis Francis, DSW
Director
Minority Fellowship Programs
Council on Social Work Education
1600 Duke Street
Alexandria, VA 22314-3421

Sarah Stanley, MS, RN
Senior Policy Analyst
American Nurses Association
600 Maryland Avenue, SW
Suite 100 West
Washington, DC 20024-2571

Foreword

Although psychologists are often the most highly trained mental health providers in rural areas, their numbers are often small. Learning to work with other mental health providers in a community context presents an opportunity for them to increase the availability of mental health and substance abuse services. Interdisciplinary approaches to the delivery of mental health and substance abuse services are an important way that the existing providers in rural areas can ensure that rural residents have access to these services. The American Psychological Association Rural Health Task Force, chaired by Michael Enright, PhD, conceived of the project described in this report in response to the perceived need for psychologists working in rural areas to maximize their effectiveness in delivering mental health and substance abuse services. The project was developed in response to a Request for Proposals from the Bureau of Health Professions of the Health Resources and Services Administration and was supported by their contract #240-BHPr-10(2). The proposal for the contract was developed in collaboration with the American Nurses Association and the Council on Social Work Education.

Russ Newman, PhD, JD
Executive Director
APA Practice Directorate

Acknowledgments

This curriculum has been a collaborative effort involving many individuals and groups who provided knowledge and hard work to accomplish the many complex tasks to produce it. The members of the Planning and Advisory Task Force listed on page v worked with determination over a period of 18 months to accomplish this truly interdisciplinary effort. Meetings of the Task Force were held at the University of Utah in Salt Lake City. The cooperation and support of the Department of Educational Psychology, the College of Nursing, and the School of Social Work of the University played a major role in the meetings' success. The work of the Task Force benefited from the review and comments of the APA Rural Health Task Force whose members are listed on page vi. The management of the project was facilitated by a Project Management Committee whose membership is listed on page vi.

This publication was edited by Sarah J. Trembath of APA Books. The Director of the Office of Rural Health in the APA Practice Directorate, Gil Hill, served as Project Director. He was ably assisted by Marquette W. Turner, Program Assistant in the Office of Rural Health. Project officers for the American Nurses Association and the Council on Social Work Education were Sarah Stanley, MS, RN, and E. Aracelis Francis, DSW. This publication is a collaborative effort of the three associations.

Russ Newman, PhD, JD
Executive Director
APA Practice Directorate

I

Introduction

A. Mental Health in Rural America

Gauging the overall mental health of rural America is a task made difficult by the general lack of current, reliable studies on the prevalence of mental disorders in rural residents. What little data there are seem to indicate that the prevalence of mental disorders in rural Americans is similar to that of their urban counterparts. Notable differences between the two communities exist, however, both in the availability of mental health care and in the prevalence of specific disorders.

Numerous studies have found strong positive correlations between the mental and economic health of rural communities. Not surprisingly, economic crises apparently contributed to mental health problems in rural communities. The result of this is reflected in numerous studies that record the increased incidence of certain mental disorders. Among those families forced to leave their farms, nearly all adults experienced some depression with the majority experiencing prolonged depression. State-supported mental health services such as suicide prevention, education, and support groups, and individual counseling have waned. Furthermore, other sources of services (e.g., nonprofit foundations and private practitioners) are less available in rural areas.

The most recent examination of the data on mental health and substance abuse problems in rural areas is contained in a monograph published by Wagenfeld, Murray, Mohatt, and Debruyn (1994). Chapters 2 and 3 discuss available data on these subjects. The need for additional efforts to gather better rural data is reinforced.

A significant handicap for rural mental health care providers is the lack of acceptance and awareness of both mental health care providers and problems within the rural community. In a recent American Psychological Association (APA) survey of professionals serving rural youth, the majority of respondents felt that people in rural areas were not aware of how they could benefit from such services or of how to obtain them. Moreover, only one fifth of the professionals felt that the youth they serve often believe in and/or confide in their mental health care providers.

Like primary health care practitioners, mental health professionals in rural areas face problems in having fewer training opportunities, fewer colleagues with whom to consult, and more diverse demands placed upon them than do their urban counterparts. And as in urban environments, primary care physicians provide much of the mental health care, but they receive little training in mental health diagnosis and treatment.

The problems with quality, access, and understanding of mental health care in rural areas suggest that promoting interdisciplinary training of psychologists, nurses, and social workers is vitally important. The need becomes clearer when considering that many of the behavior related problems afflicting the rural community are amenable to proven prevention and treatment strategies that are best provided by trained mental health care professionals. Interdisciplinary team training will facilitate health and mental health clinics sharing a single service site and routine consultation between groups. Social workers, psychologists, clinical psychiatric nurse specialists, and paraprofessionals play an important role in extending rural mental health services to those in need. Linkage of these services can provide better utilization of existing mental health care personnel, increase awareness and understanding of mental health services, and contribute to overall health in rural areas.

B. Implementing the Curriculum

Although this curriculum could be viewed as "one size fits all," it is the intention of the developers that the curriculum be tailored to recognize the strengths of each rural site that uses it, the needs of the site, the demographics of the site, and participating personnel. The curriculum was developed to address the mental health needs of Jackson, Wyoming; Las Vegas, New Mexico; and Lame Deer, Montana, with the hope that it can be adapted and applied in other rural communities as well.

Glossary

AFRICAN AMERICAN United States citizens who are of African descent.

AMERICAN INDIAN United States citizens who are descended from the indigenous peoples of the North American continent.

COMMUNITY A group of people residing in the same locality under the same government.

CULTURAL COMPETENCE A set of academic and interpersonal skills that allow individuals to increase their understanding and appreciation of cultural differences and similarities within, among, and between groups. This requires a willingness and an ability to draw on community based values, traditions, and customs to work with persons of and from the community in developing interventions, communications, and other points.

CULTURAL SENSITIVITY An awareness of the nuances of one's own culture and other cultures.

CULTURE The shared values, norms, traditions, customs, arts, history, folklore, and institutions of a group of people.

ETHNIC Belonging to a common group often linked by race, nationality, and language with a common cultural heritage and/or derivation.

ETHNICITY Affiliation with an ethnic group.

FRONTIER A low population density land area (e.g., county), which has six or fewer persons per square mile. People living in these areas can have severe problems with access to health care.

HISPANIC A general term used to refer to persons of Spanish American descent living in the United States (e.g., Cuban, Mexican, and Puerto Rican/Americans), who may share a common language and some cultural values. However, they are not a homogenous group.

INTERDISCIPLINARY An integrated approach in which various disciplines work together in the diagnosis and treatment of patients.

MINORITY A racial, religious, political, national, or other group thought to be different from the larger group of which it is a part.

MULTICULTURAL Composed of more than one culture.

MULTIDISCIPLINARY Various disciplines belonging to a clinical group, who practice in a parallel manner.

NATIVE AMERICAN People who are descended from the indigenous populations of the western hemisphere.

PRACTICUM A supervised clinical experience during which one implements didactic study in a clinical setting.

RURAL A multitude of definitions exist (see chapter 1, "Defining Rural," in *National Rural Health Policy Atlas* for a thorough discussion). The Census Bureau definition of a rural population includes all those people living outside of 1) urban areas that are named, or 2) incorporated places with 2,500 or more residents. It is important to understand that rural residents generally have shared beliefs and values that are somewhat different than those found in urban areas.

This curriculum has been designed to be taught by an interdisciplinary team consisting of a psychologist, a nurse, and a social worker. Obviously, the portions of the curriculum dealing with interdisciplinary team-building for treatment also apply to teaching, so the faculty's familiarity with the literature and subject matter is essential for implementation.

Students should also be selected from psychology, nursing, and social work. Of course, the inclusion of additional professionals, such as primary care physicians, should also be considered if they are present at the target site. The curriculum developers anticipated that adjustments would be made in the conduct of training to suit the education level of students.

An excellent Annenberg CPB videotape series with accompanying manuals entitled "Rural Communities: Legacy and Change" has been produced and is a useful adjunct to the teaching of the curriculum.[1]

C. Objectives of the Curriculum

Curriculum objectives are to provide students with the following skills that will enable them to provide effective mental health services in rural areas:

1. Assess community needs.
2. Identify community and professional resources.

[1]For ordering information, call 1-800-LEARNER.

3. Build interdisciplinary teams.
4. Resolve interdisciplinary/interagency conflicts.
5. Develop and improve existing interdisciplinary mental health/substance abuse (MH/SA) service delivery.
6. Conduct evaluations of interdisciplinary MH/SA service delivery programs.
7. Conceptualize and implement all of the above in a culturally competent manner.

II

Preliminary Seminars

A. Rural Culture and History

Goals

1. Identify and discuss the social, economic, political, and religious influences affecting rural communities.
2. Understand the importance of ethnic and cultural influences in rural communities and the importance of oral tradition.
3. Recognize the uniqueness of each region and community. Identify types of problems, their contexts, and related data and information.

Resources

Bicknell, E. H. (1991). A rural community-based model for care delivery to chronically mentally ill elderly. In Bushy, A. (Ed.), *Rural nursing: Volume II* (53–55). Newbury Park, CA: Sage.

Buckwater, K., Abraham, L., Smith, M., & Smillin, D. (1993). Nursing outreach to rural elderly people who are mentally ill. *Hospital & Community Psychiatry, 44* (9), 821–823.

Bushy, A. (1991). *Rural nursing: Volume II.* Newbury Park, CA: Sage.

Collins, A., & Pancoast, D. L. (1976). *Natural helping networks.* Washington, DC: NASW Press.

Davidson, O. G. (1990). *Broken heartland: The rise of America's rural ghetto.* New York: Free Press.

Farley, O. W., Griffiths, K. A., Fraser, M., & Jorgensen, L. B. (1988). Rural social work: Addressing the crisis of rural America. In J. S. McNeil and S. E. Weinstein (Eds.), *Innovations in health care practice* (pp. 50–97). Washington, DC: NASW Press.

Farley, O. W., Griffiths, K. A., Skidmore, R. A., & Thackeray, M. G. (1982). *Rural social work practice.* New York: Free Press.

Fitchen, J. (1991). *Endangered spaces enduring places: Change, identity, and survival in rural America.* Boulder, CO: Westview.

Ginsberg, L. (Ed.). (in press). *Social work in rural communities* (2nd ed.). Alexandria, VA: Council of Social Work Education.

Hall, E. T. (1959). *The silent language.* Greenwich, CT: Fawcett.

Lee, H. J. (1991). Definitions of rural: A review of the literature. In A. Bushy (Ed.), *Rural nursing: Volume II* (pp. 7–20). Newbury Park, CA: Sage.

Skidmore, R. A., Thackeray, M. G., & Farley, O. W. (1991). *Introduction to social work* (pp. 304–310). Englewood Cliffs, NJ: Prentice Hall.

Vidich, A., & Bensmann, J. (1968). *Small town in mass society: Class, power and religion in a rural community.* Garden City, NJ: Anchor.

Wagenfield, M. O., Murray, J. D., Mohatt, D. F., & Debruyn, J. C. (1994). *Mental health and rural America: 1980–1993.* Rockville, MD: Health Resources and Services Administration.

B. Rural Mental Health and Substance Abuse Problems

Goals

1. Understand epidemiological terms and the language of defining MH/SA health status.
2. Understand the impact of HIV/AIDS in rural areas.
3. Understand the unique aspects of women's mental health issues in rural areas.
4. Review the existing literature on rural mental health and substance abuse problems and how they are defined within the different disciplines.
5. Identify the perception and attitudes toward mental health, substance abuse, and HIV/AIDS and their treatment in rural communities.
6. Recognize barriers to service delivery and access to MH/SA care, and the role of the interdisciplinary team.

In addition to mental health and substance abuse problems per se, there are two important issues that must be examined while finding solutions to rural community mental health problems: HIV/AIDS and women's mental health.

In July of 1990, the Department of Health and Human Services' (DHHS) Office of Rural Health Policy and the Associate Administrator for AIDS convened an invitational workshop titled "HIV Infection in Rural Areas: Issues in Prevention and Services." Workshop participants identified a set of guiding principles addressing denial: "In many rural communities, there is denial that HIV disease is a problem that must be addressed." The workshop developed recommendations to the secretary of DHHS in five categories that cut across health care and prevention activities. Lam and Liu (1994) identified a second wave of the AIDS epidemic in the 1980s as taking place in rural areas:

> On the basis of our national AIDS data by county for 1982–1990, we have confirmed that AIDS prevalence is rising rapidly in rural America. Such a dangerous trend is expected to continue in the next decade of the AIDS pandemic. Together with other sobering trends of steady increase among the hetrosexual population, low-income classes, and ethnic minority groups, the AIDS pandemic has gained deeper and more troublesome roots in the populations where medical facilities are generally less available and in rural areas. (p. 490)

Rural women are resilient and seem to find rural life satisfying and meaningful (Striegel, 1994), but multiple risk factors are present in the rural community. Delworth, Veach, and Grohe (1988) discuss stressors for farm women such as invisibility and role overload. The roles of farm women have been changing from a focus on emotional support for the family to one in which the farm woman has more responsibilities. The farm crisis of the 1980s increased financial stressors and affected rural women's work contributions. These contributions include both on-farm labor and off-farm employment. In addition, the farm woman is taking a greater part in important decision-making on the farm. In addition to these added contributions, she maintains her original roles of mother, housekeeper, and emotional supporter. In spite of her new contributions, the farm woman remains an unacknowledged and invisible asset because cultural norms still define her solely as emotional caretaker of farm and family. These women have feelings of guilt and shame because of conflict between traditional values and expectations and the reality of their lives. They are also under stress because they tend to ignore their own needs in order to support the needs of family and farm.

Delworth et al. (1988) also outlined a model for assessment and intervention for rural women. This approach discusses stressors and conflicts for three general value orientations for farm women: traditional orientation, conflicted orientation, and emerging orientation. Clinical implications for each group are discussed.

Rural women are also at risk because of difficulties seeking help for problems (Kreitlow, 1988). Their traditional values and a belief that they should be able to solve their problems alone prolongs their difficulties and influences the type of help finally sought. Clergy and family are preferred to mental health professionals.

Resources

Achenbach, T., Howell, C. T., Quay, H. C., & Conners, H. C. (1991). National survey of problems and competencies among 4–16 year olds: Parents' reports for normative and clinical samples. *Monographs of the Society for Research in Child Development, 6* (3, Serial No. 225).

Adams, R. D., & Benjamin, M. L. (1988). Innovative approaches to mental health service delivery in rural areas. *Journal of Rural Community Psychology, 9* (2), 41–50.

Armstrong, P. S., & Schulman, M. D. (1990). Financial strain and depression among farm operators: The role of perceived economic hardship and personal control. *Rural Sociology, 55* (4), 475–493.

Baclacki, M. F. (1988). Assessing mental health needs in the rural community: A critique of assessment approaches. *Issues in Mental Health Nursing, 9,* 299–315.

Barrett, J. (1987). *Mending a broken heartland.* Alexandria, VA: Capitol.

Barrett, J. E., Barrett, J. A., Oxman, T. E., & Gerber, P. D. (1988). The prevalence of psychiatric disorders in a primary care practice. *Archives of General Psychiatry, 45,* 1100–1106.

Barsky, A. J., & Klerman, G. L. (1983). Overview: Hypochondriasis, bodily complaints and somatic styles. *American Journal of Psychiatry, 140,* 273–283.

Beeson, P. G., & Johnson, D. R. (1987, May). *A panel study of change (1981–1986) in rural mental health status: Effects of the rural crisis.* Paper presented at the NIMH National Conference on Mental Health Statistics, Denver, CO. (Available from: Dr. Peter G. Beeson, Nebraska Department of Public Institutions, P.O. Box 94728, Lincoln, NE 68588.)

Beeson, P. G., Johnson, D. R., & Ortega, S. T. (1991). *The farm crisis and mental health: A longitudinal (1981, 1986, 1989) and comparative study of the economy and mental health status.* Unpublished manuscript. (Available from: Dr. Peter G. Beeson, Nebraska Department of Public Institutions, P.O. Box 94728, Lincoln, NE 68588.)

Bender, L. D., Green, B. L., Hady, T. F., Kuehn, J. A., Nelson, J. R., Perkinson, L., & Ross, P. J. (1985, September). *The diverse social and economic structure of nonmetropolitan America.* (Rural Development Research Report No. 49.) Washington, DC: Economic Research Service, U.S. Department of Agriculture.

Blazer, D., Crowell, B. A., & George, L. R. (1987). Alcohol abuse and dependence in the rural South. *Archives of General Psychiatry, 44,* 736–740.

Blazer, D., Crowell, B. A., George, L. K., & Landerman, R. (1986). Urban/rural differences in depressive disorders: Does age make a difference? In J. E. Barrett & R. N. Rose (Eds.), *Mental disorders in the community: Progress and challenge* (pp. 32–46). New York: Guilford.

Blazer, D., George, L. K., Landerman, R., Pennybacker, M., Melville, M. L., Woodbury, M., Manton, K. G., Jordan, K., & Locke, B. Z. (1985). Psychiatric disorders: A rural/urban comparison. *Archives of General Psychiatry, 42,* 653–656.

Blazer, D., Hughes, D., & George, L. K. (1987). Stressful life events and the onset of a generalized anxiety syndrome. *American Journal of Psychiatry, 144,* 1178–1183.

Blazer, D., Swartz, M., Woodbury, M., Manton, K. G., Hughes, D., & George, L. K. (1988). Depressive symptoms and depressive diagnoses in a community population. *Archives of General Psychiatry, 45*, 1078–1084.

Boyd, J. H., Weissman, M. M., Thompson, W. D., & Myers, J. K. (1982). Screening for depression in a community sample: Understanding the discrepancies between depression symptom and diagnostic scales. *Archives of General Psychiatry, 39*, 1195–1204

Boyd, M. A. (1992). The individual who is severely and persistently mentally ill: Directions for research and practice. *Issues in Mental Health Nursing, 13*, 207–208.

Bultena, G., Lasley, P., & Geller, J. (1986). The farm crisis: Patterns and impacts of financial distress among Iowa farm families. *Rural Sociology, 5* (14), 436–448.

Chavetz, L., & Barnes, L. (1989). Issues in psychiatric caregiving. *Archives of Psychiatric Nursing, 3* (4), 61–68.

Christopherson, V. A., Escher, M. R., & Bainton, B. R. (1984). Reasons for drinking among the elderly in rural Arizona. *Journal of Studies on Alcohol, 45*, 417–423.

Ciarlo, J. A., & Tweed, D. L. (1992, November). *Exploring Colorado's need for mental health services: Some preliminary findings*. Paper presented to the meeting of the American Evaluation Association, Seattle, WA.

Cohen, S., Ramarck, T., & Mermelstein, R. (1983). A global measure of perceived stress. *Journal of Health and Social Behavior, 24*, 385–396.

"Coming to the Country." Videotape available from the Great Plains Staff Training and Development for Rural Mental Health, Department of Psychology, 304 Burnett Hall, Lincoln, NE 68588-0375.

Cooper, J. (1994). Country music launches AIDS campaign in rural areas. *Broadcasting & Cable, 124* (1), 55.

Coulam, R. F., Hargrove, D. S., & Lentner, T. H. (1991). NIMH-funded rural mental health demonstration projects. Technical assistance report. *Rural Community Mental Health Newsletter, 17* (2), 1–16.

Davis, K. A., et al. (1992). Moving home to live: Migration of HIV-infected persons to rural states. *Journal of the Association of Nurses in AIDS Care, 3* (4), 42.

Delworth, U., Veach, S. D., & Grohe, L. (1988). Clinical issues with farm women. In P. A. Keller & S. R. Heyman (Eds.), *Innovations in clinical practice: A source book.* (pp. 423–431). Sarasota, FL: Professional Resource Exchange.

De Nitto, D. (1982). Alcoholism and rural America. *Human services in the rural environment, 7*, 3–9.

Diclemente, R. J., Brown, L. K., Beausoleil, N. I., et al. (1993). Comparison of AIDS knowledge and HIV - related sexual risk behaviors among adolescents in low and high AIDS prevalence. *Journal of Adolescent Health, 14* (3), 231–236

Diclemente, R. J. (1990). Adolescents' HIV related knowledge, attitudes and behavior. (Cassette recording from 12th Annual Adolescent Health Care Conference: Adolescents and AIDS). Minneapolis, MN: University of Minnesota Continuing Medical Education.

Dohrenwend, B. P., & Dohrenwend, B. S. (1982). Perspectives on the past and future of psychiatric epidemiology. *American Journal of Public Health, 72*, 1271–1279.

Dohrenwend, B. P., & Dohrenwend, B. S. (1971). *The prevalence of psychiatric disorders in urban versus rural settings*. Proceedings of the Fifth World Congress of Psychiatry, Mexico City.

Farley, et al. (1982). *Rural social work practice* (pp. 191–201). New York: Free Press.

Francell, C. G., Conn, V. S., & Gray, D. P. (1988). Families' perceptions of burden of care for chronic mentally ill relatives. *Hospital and Community Psychiatry, 39*, 1296–1300.

Furman, L. E., & Selby, A. (1982). Rural alcoholic women: Study and treatment. *Human Services in the Rural Environment, 7*, 15–23.

Gallagher, E., & Delworth, U. (1993). The third shift: Juggling employment, family, and the farm. *Journal of Rural Community Psychology, 12* (2), 21–36

George, L. K., Hughes, D. R., & Blazer, D. G. (1986). Urban/rural differences in the prevalence of anxiety disorders. *The American Journal of Social Psychiatry, 6*, 249–258.

Gibbons, S., Wylie, M. L., Echterling, D., & French, J. (1986). Patterns of alcohol use among rural and small-town adolescents. *Adolescence, 21*, 887–900.

Health Services Admininstration. (1991, April). *HIV infection in rural areas: Issues in prevention and services; an invitational workshop.* Rockville, MD: Health Services Administration.

Heffernan, J. B., & Heffernan, W. D. (1985, May). *The effects of the agricultural crisis on the health and lives of farm families.* Statement prepared for a hearing before members of the Committee on Agriculture, U.S. House of Representatives, Washington, DC.

Hermelstein, J., & Sundet, P. (1986). Rural community mental health centers' response to the farm crisis. *Human Services in the Rural Environment, 10,* 21–26.

Holloway, T. (1990). *Syphilis, crack and AIDS: Rural Georgia's new epidemic.* Waycross, GA: Georgia Department of Human Services.

Hoyt, D. R. (1988, October). *Economic stress and mental health in rural Iowa.* Prepared for the Iowa Department of Human Services. (Available from D. R. Hoyt, Department of Sociology, Iowa State University, Ames, IA 50011.)

Husaini, B. A., & Neff, J. A. (1982). The prevalence of psychopathology in rural Tennessee and Oklahoma. In P. A. Keller & J. D. Murray (Eds.), *Handbook of rural community mental health* (pp. 45–51). New York: Human Sciences Press.

International Institute of Rural Reconstruction. (1992). *Participatory approach to rural AIDS education: A workshop manual.* New York: Author.

Kane, D. F., DiMartino, E., & Jimenez, J. (1990). Short-term multifamily groups for relatives coping with chronic schizophrenia. *Archives of Psychiatric Nursing, 6* (6), 343–353.

Kellner, R. (1985). Functional somatic complaints and hypochondriasis. *Archives of General Psychiatry, 48,* 821–833.

Kessler, R. C. (1990, Winter). The national comorbidity survey, *DIS Newsletter,* pp. 1–2.

Kiger, G., & Riley, P. J. (1988, August). *The relationship between community integration and mental health in rural areas.* Paper presented to Rural Sociological Society, Athens, GA.

Kreitlow, B. (1988, December 27). Rural women less likely to seek social services help: University of Iowa Study. *Cedar Rapids Gazette,* C6.

Lam, N.S.-N., & Liu, K-B. (1994). Spread of AIDS in rural America, 1982–1990. *Journal of Acquired Immune Deficiency Syndromes, 7,* 485–490.

Lantz, A., Sackett, K., & Halpern, J. (1980). Alcohol-related problems in rapidly-growing communities. In J. A. Davenport & J. Davenport, III (Eds.), *Boom towns: Problems and promises in the energy vortex* (pp. 71–83). Laramie: University of Wyoming.

Lassey, M. L., & Carlson, J. E. (1979). Drinking among teenagers: Rural-urban comparison in peer influence. *Journal of Alcohol and Drug Education, 24,* 8–18.

Linn, J. G., & Husaini, B. A. (1987). Determinants of psychological depression and coping behaviors of Tennessee farm residents. *Journal of Community Psychology, 15,* 503–512.

Lyson, T. A. (1986). Who cares about the farmer? Apathy and the current farm crisis. *Rural Sociology, 51* (4), 490–502.

Martinez-Brawley, E. (1987). Rural social work. In A. Minahan (Ed.), *Encyclopedia of social work* (18th ed.). Silver Spring, MD: NASW Press.

Martinez-Brawley, E. (1990). *Perspectives on the small community: Humanistic views for practitioners.* Washington, DC: NASW Press.

Maurin, J. T., & Boyd, C. (Eds.). (1990). Burden of mental illness on the family: A critical review. *Archives of Psychiatric Nursing, 4* (2), 99–107.

McKinley, A. (1991). Suicide among the rural elderly: An Arizona perspective. In A. Bushey (Ed.), *Rural nursing: Volume II* (pp. 297–308). Newbury Park, CA: Sage.

Miller, W. A., Qualteere-Bucher, P., & Lauber, C., et al. (1990). AIDS knowledge and attitudes among adolescents in the rural Southwest. The *Journal of Rural Health, 6* (3), 246–255.

Mirowsky, J., & Ross, C. E. (1989). *Social causes of psychological distress. New York: Aldine de Gruyter. National Institute of Mental Health. (1986). Summary report on policy forum on rural stress.* Unpublished report. Rockville, MD: Office of Policy Analysis Development.

Montana Office of Public Instruction, AIDS Education Program Curriculum Services Unit. (1990). *Guidelines to communicable disease control policies in Montana schools: A guide and model policy for communicable diseases including HIV infected students and staff.* Helena, MT: Author.

Montana State University. (1992). *AIDS: A rural perspective.* Bozeman, MT: Author.

Napier, T. L., Bachtel, D. C., & Carter, M. V. (1983). Factors associated with illegal drug use in rural Georgia. *Journal of Drug Education, 13,* 119–140.

National AIDS Support Center. (1992). *Rural community AIDS Journal* (2nd ed.). Santa Fe, NM: Author.

National Association of State Alcohol and Drug Abuse Directors. (1990). *AIDS policy seminar on issues for rural areas and states with a low incidence of HIV/AIDS associated with substance abuse: Indianapolis, IN.* Washington, DC: Author.

National Mental Health Association. (1989). *Report of the national action commission on the mental health of rural Americans.* Alexandria, VA: Author.

Neff, J. A. (1984). Race differences in psychological distress: The effects of sex, urbanicity, and measurement strategy. *American Journal of Community Psychology, 12,* 337–357.

Neff, J. A., & Husaini, B. A. (1987). Urbanicity, race, and psychological distress. *Journal of Community Psychology, 15,* 520–536.

Patton, L. (1989). Setting the rural health services research agenda: The congressional perspective. *HSR: Health Services Research, 23,* 1005–1051.

Regier, D. A., Myers, J. K., Framer, M., Robins, L. N., Blazer, D., Hough, R., Eaton, W., & Locke, B. (1984). The NIMH epidemiologic catchment area program: Historical context, major objectives, and study population characteristics. *Archives of General Psychiatry, 41,* 934–941.

Rettig, R. D., Bauer, J. W., & Danes, S. M. (1990). *Adjustment of farm families to economic stress: A two-year study.* (Minnesota Report 220 -1990, Item No. AD-MR-3994). St. Paul, MN: Minnesota Agricultural Experiment Station.

Robins, L., Helzer, J., Croughan, J., & Ratcliff, K. (1981). National Institute of Mental Health Diagnostic Interview Schedule: Its history, characteristics and validity. *Archives of General Psychiatry, 38,* 381–389.

Robins, L., Locke, B. Z., & Regier, D. A. (1991). An overview of psychiatric disorders in America. In L. N. Robins & D. A. Regier (Eds.), *Psychiatric disorders in America* (pp. 328–366). New York: Free Press.

Robins, L. N., & Regier, D. A. (Eds.). (1991). *Psychiatric disorders in America.* New York: Free Press.

Robins, L. N., Tipp, J., & Przybeck, T. (1991). Antisocial personality. In L. N. Robins & D. A. Regier (Eds.), *Psychiatric disorders in America* (pp. 258–290). New York: Free Press.

Robins, L. N., Wing, J., Wittchen, H. U., Helzer, J. E., Babor, T. F., Burke, J., Farmer, A., Jablenski, A., Oickens, R., Regier, D. A., Sartorius, N., & Tallowy, L. H. (1988). The composite international diagnostic interview. *Archives of General Psychiatry, 45,* 1069–1077.

Rosenblatt, P. C. (1991). *Farming is in our blood: Farm families in economic crisis.* Ames, IA: Iowa State University.

Sacramento AIDS Foundation & Center for AIDS Research, Education and Services. (1990). *HIV 2000: A guide to planning for HIV care in Northern California.* Sacramento, CA: Author.

Sarvela, P. D., & McClendon, E. J. (1988). Indicators of rural drug use. *Journal of Youth and Adolescence, 17,* 335–347.

Sarvela, P. D., Pape, D. J., & Bajracharya, S. M. (1990a). Age of first use of drugs among rural midwestern youth. *Human Services in the Rural Environment, 13,* 9–15.

Sarvela, P. D., Pape, D. J., Odulana, J., & Bajracharya, S. M. (1990b). Drinking, drug use, and driving among rural midwestern youth. *Journal of School Health, 60,* 215–219.

Schulman, M. D., & Armstrong, P. S. (1989a). The farm crisis: An analysis of social psychological distress among North Carolina farm operators. *American Journal of Community Psychology, 17* (4), 423–442.

Schulman, M. D., & Armstrong, P. S. (1989b). Perceived stress, social support and survival: North Carolina farm operators and crisis. *Journal of Sociology and Social Welfare, 17* (3), 3–22.

Spitzer, R. L., Endicott, J., & Robins, E. (1975). *Research diagnostic criteria for a selected group of functional disorders.* New York: Biometrics Research, New York State Psychiatric Institute.

Stack, S. (1982). Suicide: A decade review of the sociological literature. *Deviant Behavior, 4,* 41–66.

Striegel, M. R. (1994). *Sustainability of agriculture and life satisfaction of farm women.* Master's Equivalency Project, The University of Iowa, Iowa City.

Swaim, R., Beauvais, F., Edwards, R. W., & Oetting, E. R. (1986). Adolescent drug use in three small rural communities in the Rocky Mountain region. *Journal of Drug Education, 16,* 57–73.

Swartz, M., Blazer, D., George, L. (1986). Somatization disorder in a community population. *American Journal of Psychiatry, 143,* 1403–1408.

Swartz, M., Landerman, R., Blazer, D., & George, L. (1989). Somatization symptoms in the community: A rural/urban comparison. *Psychosomatics, 30,* 44–53.

United Way of Butte/Glenn Counties. (1993). *Coming home guide for HIV Affected persons.* [Brochure].

University of Utah Health Behavior Laboratory Research and Evaluation Program. (1991). *Montana Youth Risk Behavior Survey.* Helena, MT: Montana Office of Public Intervention, AIDS Education Program Curriculum Services Unit.

U.S. General Accounting Office (1990). *Rural drug abuse: Prevalence, relation to crime, and programs.* (GAO/PEMD - 90 - 24). Washington, DC: U.S. Government Printing Office.

U.S. Congress, Departments of Labor, Health and Human Services, and Education and related agencies appropriations. (1986). Senate Report 99-408 (to accompany H.R. 5233).

U.S. Congress, Office of Technology Assessment. (1990, September.) *Health care (OTA-H-434).* Washington, DC: U.S. Government Printing Office.

U.S. Department of Health and Human Services. (1990, July). *HIV infection in rural areas: Issues in prevention and services.* Report of an invitational workshop. Washington, DC: Author.

Vaillant, G. E., & Schnurr, P. (1988). What is a case? *Archives of General Psychiatry, 45,* 313–319.

Wagenfeld, M. O. (1982). Psychopathology in rural areas: Issues and evidence. In P. A. Keller & J. D. Murray (Eds.), *Handbook of Rural Community Mental Health* (pp. 30–44). New York: Human Sciences.

Wagenfeld, N. O., Goldsmith, H. F., Stiles, D., Longest, J., & Nanderscheid, R. W. *Inpatient mental health services: An intraregional comparison.* Manuscript submitted for publication.

Walker, J. L., & Walker, L. J. S. (1988). Self-reported stress symptoms in farmers. *Journal of Clinical Psychology, 44* (1), 10–16.

Warheit, G., Holzer, C. E., & Arey, S. A. (1975). Race and mental illness: An epidemiologic update. *Journal of Health and Social Behavior, 16,* 243–256.

Weibel-Orlando, J., Weisner, T., and Long, J. (1984). Urban and rural Indian drinking patterns: Implications for intervention policy development. *Substance Abuse and Alcohol Actions/Misuse, 5,* 45–57.

Weissman, M. M., Bruce, M. L., Leaf, P. J., Florio, L. P., & Holzer, C. III (1991). Affective disorders. In L. N. Robins and D. A. Regier (Eds.), *Psychiatric disorders in America* (pp. 53-80). New York: Free Press.

Weisz, R. (1979). Stress and mental health in a boom town. In J. A. Davenport & J. Davenport, III. (Eds.), *The boom town and human services* (pp. 31–47). Laramie: University of Wyoming.

Wilkinson, K. P., & Israel, J. D. (1984). Suicide and rurality in urban society. *Suicide and Life-Threatening Behavior, 14,* 187–199.

Windle, C. (1991). *The other depression in rural areas.* Presentation to the National Rural Electric Cooperative Association Directors Conference, Nashville, TN. Rockville, MD: Division of Biometry and Applied Services, National Institute of Mental Health.

Winfree, L. T., Theis, H. E., & Griffiths, C. T. (1981). Drug use in rural America: A cross-cultural examination of complementary social deviance theories. *Youth and Society, 12,* 465–489.

Zahner, G. E. P., Jacobs, J. H., Freeman, D. H., & Trainor, K. F. (in press). Rural-urban child psychopathology in a northeastern U.S. state: 1986-1989. *Journal of the American Academy of Child and Adolescent Psychiatry.*

C. Relationship of Ethnic Culture to Rural Mental Health Services

Goals

1. Understand the impact of the interaction between social institutions and ethnicity on the delivery of mental health services.
2. Recognize the impact of the provider's own culture, sensitivity, and awareness as it affects his or her ability to deliver MH/SA care.
3. Understand alternative treatment sources in the ethnic minority culture.

Resources

Bean, S. (1989). Indian child welfare social policy history module. In E. Gonzalez-Santin & A. Lewis (Eds.), *Collaboration: The key* (pp. 29–49). Tempe: Arizona State University, School of Social Work.

Bertold, S. M. (1989). Spiritism as a form of psychotherapy: Implications for social work practice. *Social Casework, 70,* 502–509.

Broman, C. L. (1987). Race differences in professional help seeking. *American Journal of Community Psychology, 15,* 473–489.

Castle, E. N. (1985). The forgotten hinterlands: Rural America. *Annual Report 1986* (pp. 2–10). Washington, DC: Resources for the Future.

Cole, J., & Pilisuk, M. (1976). Differences in the provision of mental health services by race. *American Journal of Orthopsychiatry, 46,* 510–525.

Comos Diaz, L., & Minrath, M. (1985). Psychotherapy with ethnic minority borderline clients. *Psychotherapy: Theory, research, & practice, 22* (2), 418–426.

Draguns, J. G. (1984). Assessing mental health and disorders across cultures. In P. B. Pedersen, N. Sartorius, & A. J. Marsella (Eds.). *Mental health services: The cross-cultural context* (pp. 199–220). Beverly Hills, CA: Sage.

DuBray, W. H. (1985). American Indian values: Critical factor in coursework. *Social Coursework, 66,* 30–37.

Dufrene, P. M., & Coleman, V. D. (1982). Counseling Native Americans: Guidelines for group process. *The Journal for Specialists in Group Work, 17* (4), 229–234.

Escobar, J. I. (1987). Cross cultural aspects of the somatization trait. *Hospital and Community Psychiatry, 38,* 174–180.

Galan, F. J. (1985). Traditional values about family behavior: The case of the Chicano client. *Social Thought, 11* (3), 14–22.

Gibson, G. (1985). Chicanos and their support systems in interaction with social institutions. In M. Bloom (Ed.). *Life span development,* (2nd ed.). New York: Macmillan.

Good Tracks, J. G. (1973). Native American non-interference. *Social Work, 17* (4), 30–34.

Green, J. W. (1992). Language and cross-cultural social work. In J. W. Green (Ed.), *Cultural awareness in the human services* (pp. 67–83). Englewood Cliffs, NJ: Prentice-Hall.

Gupta, Giri Raj. (1993). Mental disorders: Social class, race, ethnicity, and rural and urban living. In *Sociology of Mental Health* (pp. 213–238). Boston: Allyn and Bacon.

Herring, R. D. (1992). Seeking a new paradigm: Counseling Native Americans. *Journal of Multicultural Counseling and Development, 20,* 35–43.

Horejsi, C., Craig, B. H., & Pablo, J. (1992). Reactions by Native American parents to child protection agencies: Cultural and community factors. *Child Welfare, 59* (2), 329–342.

Javier, R. A. (1989). Linguistic considerations in the treatment of bilinguals. *Psychoanalytic Psychology, 6,* 87–96.

Joe, J. R. (1989). Values. In E. Gonzalez-Santin & A. Lewis (Eds.), *Collaboration: The key* (pp. 11–27). Tempe, AZ: Arizona State University.

Kleiman, S. (1980). *Patients and healers in the context of culture.* Berkeley, CA: University of California.

Lawson, W. B. (1986). Racial and ethnic factors in psychiatric research. *Hospital and Community Psychiatry, 38,* 1186–1190.

Loring, M., & Powell, B. (1988). Gender, race, and DSM-III: A study of the objectivity of psychiatric diagnostic behavior. *Journal of Health and Social Behavior, 29,* 1186–1190.

Meinhardt, K., & Vega, W. (1987). A method for estimating underutilization of mental health services by ethnic groups. *Hospital and Community Psychiatry, 140,* 1571–1574.

Minrath, M. (1985). Breaking the race barrier: The white therapist in interracial therapy. *Journal of Psychosocial and Mental Health Nursing, 25,* 19–25.

Mukherjee, S., et al. (1983). Misdiagnosis of schizophrenia in bipolar patients: A multi-ethnic comparison. *American Journal of Psychiatry, 140,* 1571–1574.

Pinderhughes, E. (1989). *Understanding race, ethnicity, & power.* New York: Free Press.

Renfrey, G. S. (1992). Cognitive-behavior therapy and the Native American client. *Behavior Therapy, 23,* 321–340.

Roberts, R. E. (1981). Prevalence of depressive symptoms among Mexican Americans. *Journal of Nervous and Mental Disease, 169,* 213–219.

Sands, R. G. (1991). *Clinical social work practice in community mental health.* New York: Macmillian.

Snipp, C. M., & Summers, G. F. (1991). American Indians and economic poverty. In C. M. Ducan (Ed.), *Rural poverty in America.* Westport, CT: Greenwood Press.

Torrey, E. F. (1986). *Witchdoctors and psychiatrists.* New York: Harper and Row.

Trimble, J. E., Manson, S. M., Dinges, N. G., & Medicine, B. (1984). American Indians' concepts of mental health: Reflections and directions. In P. B. Pedersen, N. Sartorius, & A. J. Marsella (Eds.), *Mental health services: The cross-cultural context* (pp. 199–220). Beverly Hills, CA: Sage.

Warhiet, G. J., Vega, W. A., Auth, J. B., & Meinhardt, K. (1985). Psychiatric symptoms and dysfunctions among Anglos and Mexican Americans: An epidemiologic study. In J. R. Greenley (Ed.), *Research in community and mental health: A research annual* (pp. 2–22). Greenwich, CT: JAI Press.

Weinert, C., & Long, K. A. (1991). The theory and research base for rural nursing practice. In A. Bushey (Ed.), *Rural nursing: Volume II* (pp. 21–38). Newbury Park, CA: Sage.

Westermyer, J. (1985). Psychiatric diagnosis across cultural boundaries. *American Journal of Psychiatry, 142,* 798–805.

D. Rural Health and Mental Health Disciplines

The disciplines of psychology, nursing, and social work complement each other well; their relationship is a natural alliance. This description can be extended to include primary care physicians as well. Collaboration between professionals in these fields has been used to treat various mental and physical conditions. Such interdisciplinary collaboration is especially needed in rural areas where existing resources must be maximized in order to provide mental health services. Successful rural interdisciplinary treatment approaches (such as in geriatric care) involve psychologists, nurses, and social workers, and focus on mental health issues.

Documented team training approaches to various health and mental health problems are more common in other countries than in the United States. For example, interdisciplinary treatment involving psychology and nursing has been used in inpatient mental health treatment of children in Britain, and in France in a system of play therapy for children.

Because primary care physicians are the dominant providers of mental health care in rural areas and because they often lack specific training, interdisciplinary training programs involving psychology, nursing, and social work are needed to compensate for the lack of mental health care personnel. Interdisciplinary team training for rural mental health care provides the means to serve these communities in ways that will maximize the services provided by a limited number of personnel over a wide geographic area. Also, training that is applicable to the three professions provides better patient care and is more cost effective than separate rural mental health curricula for each.

Goals

1. Know the role and scope of practice of the various mental health providers.
2. Know the educational preparation of mental health providers.
3. Know the legal regulation of the practice of each discipline.
4. Know the ethical principles followed by the various mental health providers.

Provider Network

1. Psychologists
2. Nurses

3. Social Workers
4. Primary Care Providers: Physicians, Physician Assistants, and Nurse Practitioners

Format

- Invite representatives from as many provider groups as possible to describe and discuss their practice and experience. This could occur in a panel format.
- Develop and review a glossary of terms used by providers in their practices.

1. Psychologists

a. Definition. Psychology is both a behavioral science and a service-oriented health profession. Psychologists study behavior and work to develop a valid and reliable body of scientific knowledge based on research. As service-oriented health professionals, psychologists implement findings from research in their prevention and treatment methodologies, which aim not only to lessen the psychological suffering of the individual, but also to improve the overall condition of society.

As a part of their general training, psychologists study a basic core of knowledge that includes the biological, mental, emotional, and social bases of behavior as well as theories that account for individual differences in behavior and learning. In order to complete their training as scientist/practitioners, they are instructed in research design and methodology, statistics, psychological diagnosis and assessment, scientific and professional ethics and standards, and intervention and treatment techniques; those who provide professional services learn a variety of other skills applicable to their specialties.

Psychologists' unique training as scientist/practitioners allows them to apply their knowledge to human behavior in a variety of contexts. In doing so, they function in many roles, such as researcher, educator, diagnostician, therapist, supervisor, consultant, administrator, social interventionist, and expert witness. Psychologists respect the central importance of freedom of inquiry and expression in research, teaching, and publication. They also strive to help the public in developing informed judgments and choices concerning human behavior.

b. History. To understand the discipline of psychology one must realize that psychology has been influenced by many schools of thought. Thus, psychology's matrix is composed of disciplines such as philosophy, medicine, physics, and physiology. To understand the history of psychology as a profession in the United States one should concentrate on a multitude of events throughout its history. However, in the following there will be a brief introduction to two models of training that were significant in the developmental history of psychology as a profession.

The scientist/practitioner model was endorsed as a result of an important conference held in Boulder, Colorado in 1949. This conference brought together 41 representatives from clinical training programs to discuss issues related to doctoral training in clinical psychology. The result of these discussions led to the endorsement of the scientist/practitioner model of training, or the Boulder model. This model emphasizes the importance of training clinical psychologists in the rigors of scientific investigation and the application of psychological principles. This model of training was one of the first steps of the profession in recognizing that psychologists are not only scientists but are also practitioners.

The Boulder model has shaped psychological training since its endorsement by the committee. The majority of doctoral programs today continue to train their students in the Boulder model. However, over the last 25 years the profession has witnessed a movement that has focused on the practice of psychology. An outgrowth from this focus was the development of a professional model of training. This model is strictly structured for the practice of psychology with less emphasis on the science of psychology.

It is important to emphasize that both models of training coexist today. In addition, it is imperative to recognize that the practice of psychology continues to flourish and advance as a result of the field's continued scientific exploration of behavior and behavior change. Thus, the profession is ever evolving and expanding its knowledge base, and psychologists continue to develop a better understanding of human behavior, improve treatment methodologies, and assist in improving the health and mental health of our society. Please refer to *Milestones in Psychological Practice: 1892–1992* (American Psychological Association, 1992b) for a more detailed account.

c. **Ethics.** The APA commits its members to adhere to the APA Ethics Code and to the rules and procedures used to implement it. Psychologists and students, whether or not they are APA members, should be aware that the Ethics Code may be applied to them by state psychology boards, courts, or other public bodies.

The Ethics Code applies only to psychologists' work-related activities, that is, activities that are part of the psychologist's scientific and professional functions or that are psychological in nature. The "Ethical Principles of Psychologists and Code of Conduct" (American Psychological Association, 1992a) is composed of two sections: general principles and ethical standards.

The general principles are as follows:

1. Competence
2. Integrity
3. Professional and scientific responsibility
4. Respect for people's rights
5. Concern for others' welfare
6. Social responsibility

The ethical standards are categorized in the following groups:

1. General standards
2. Evaluation, assessments, or intervention
3. Advertising and other public statements

4. Therapy
5. Privacy and confidentiality
6. Teaching, training, supervision, research, and publishing
7. Forensic activities
8. Resolving ethical issues

Please refer to APA's (1992a) "Ethical Principles of Psychologists and Code of Conduct" for a more complete explanation of the code.

d. Current developments

1. Hospital practice. It has long been recognized that psychologists are a valuable resource in the treatment of mental disorders and psychological disturbances. However, the majority of psychologists deliver these services outside the hospital setting. Hospital settings have typically been dominated by medical professionals. Thus the medical profession has historically been reluctant to grant psychologists hospital privileges based on "turf" issues. Despite resistance from some in the medical community, many psychologists have delivered services and worked in hospital settings.

In the recent past there have been efforts to establish hospital practicing privileges in several states. Some of these efforts have met with considerable success. Psychologists' unique training prepares them to serve in many different capacities in the hospital setting. Psychologists will be able to serve not only as practitioners who possess clinical attending, assessment, and treatment privileges, but also as administrators.[1]

2. Prescription privileges. In recent years some members of the psychological profession have attempted to gain prescriptive authority through legislative efforts. The proposed prescriptive authority would be limited to the use of psychotropic medications. This is a controversial topic within psychology and outside the profession. The following article and press release discuss current initiatives in this area.

Prescription Privileges Efforts Gain Momentum: Defense Department's Pilot Training Program Produces Its First Psychologist Graduates[2]

Psychologists' quest for the privilege of prescribing psychotropic medication is intensifying, with particularly strong progress in California.

Meanwhile, a pilot pharmacology-training program for military psychologists has produced its first two graduates, who are now authorized to prescribe medications in their new military posts.

---

[1]See *A Hospital Practice Primer for Psychologists* (American Psychological Association, 1985) for a more thorough discussion.

[2]*APA Monitor* article, September 1994.

In California, a blue-ribbon panel, working with the California School of Professional Psychology (CPA), has drafted a proposed psychopharmacology training program for psychologists. The California Psychological Association hopes the proposal can help state lawmakers craft educational requirements to be included in future state legislation granting prescription privileges to psychologists, CPA officials said.

CPA has drafted a bill that would grant the privilege to prescribe certain medications, but is waiting until next year to actively seek a lawmaker to sponsor the measure, said Peggy Dudder, the association's lobbyist. The state legislature is too immersed this year in budgetary matters and the fall elections to give the CPA's bill much attention, Dudder said.

The proposed curriculum includes six months of basic training in neuroscience and psychopharmacology, said Esteban Olmedo, PhD, a professor at the California professional school. A subsequent practicum would last another year, he added.

The American Psychological Association's Committee on the Advancement of Professional Practice provided a grant for the 11-member group, which includes physicians, pharmacists, a psychiatrist and a neuroscientist.

The Military Program

The U.S. Department of Defense psychopharmacology training program has enrolled five new participants after producing its first two graduates this past summer. Navy Cmdr. John Sexton, PhD, has been assigned to supervise an inpatient psychiatric ward at Portsmouth Naval Hospital in Chesapeake, Va. Lt. Morgan Sammons, PhD, has been stationed at the National Naval Medical Center in Bethesda, Md.

Congress in 1991 directed the Defense Department to launch the training for military psychologists interested in prescribing psychotropic medications within the military health-care system. Earlier this year, the program opened up to civilian psychologists who will serve five years of active duty in exchange for the training.

Sammons and Sexton went through three years of training, but the current program has been tailored to make it better suited for training psychologists to prescribe. The five new participants will train for only two years.

The National Outlook

At the national level, APA's CAPP has created a task force to help the committee plot a broad strategy around prescription privileges. The task force will explore the state and national efforts under way and try to weld them into a coordinated strategy, said Dan Egli, PhD, chair of the group.

The prescription-privilege issue has engendered considerable debate within psychology. Many practitioners say prescription privileges would alter psychology's scope of practice, creating a cadre of "junior psychiatrists." But support for the privilege is growing within the profession, and, if APA does not begin to deal with what is happening in the field, the organization will find itself being pulled along with no control or input, said officials in APA's Practice Directorate. As many as 25 states have task forces exploring the possibility of securing prescription authority.

California is clearly in front on the prescription-privileges drive, but other states are also making significant progress, said Pat DeLeon, PhD, recording secretary for the APA Board of Directors and a leading advocate for prescription privileges. Psychologists in Hawaii and Missouri are developing model curricula that could be incorporated into future legislation, he noted. The profession will have a stronger chance of arriving at a positive result through better coordination of efforts, said Russ Newman, PhD, JD, the directorate's executive director.

Adding some well-rounded insight to the prescription effort is Joe Pachman, PhD, MD, who is trained in psychology and preventive medicine. Pachman, of Weston, Conn., serves on the California blue-ribbon panel and the CAPP task force.

Psychiatry, which has vehemently opposed expanding prescription privileges to psychologists, will evolve into a new model of care as psychology merges into the prescription realm, Pachman predicts. Psychiatrists are already focusing more on biological aspects of mental disorders, and will continue to merge into primary-care activities, Pachman said.

Meanwhile, psychologists' emphasis on behavior fits well with prescribing, especially because compliance is often a problem among patients taking psychotropic drugs, Pachman said.

"Being a good psychopharmacologist is much more than prescribing the best medication," he said. "It's developing a therapeutic relationship so the benefits from the medications are maximized."

Two Civilian Psychologists Affiliated With the American Psychological Association Selected for DoD Psychopharmacology Demonstration Project[3]

WASHINGTON—Last week, a staff member and a congressional fellow from the American Psychological Association (APA) were sworn into the U.S. Army in order to begin a psychopharmacology post-doctoral fellowship next month. These two psychologists, along with three military psychologists, were selected for the 1994–1996 fellowship. This is the first year this fellowship was offered to properly credentialed civilian practitioners on the condition that they enter active duty as an officer in the U.S. Army.

This Department of Defense fellowship, known as the Psychopharmacology Demonstration Project (PDP), is a congressionally mandated two-year fellowship designed to prepare military clinical psychologists to be credentialed to prescribe psychotropic medications independently within the Department of Defense Health Care System. The 1994–96 fellowship will be the third iteration of this project. Two fellows will graduate from the first iteration this month, and two additional fellows are in their first year of the fellowship.

Anita Brown, Ph.D., is currently an assistant executive director for education at the American Psychological Association, and Debra Dunivin, Ph.D, is completing her second year as an APA Congressional Fellow. Dr. Brown,

[3]APA press release, June 17, 1994.

who has worked for three years at APA, was a lecturer in psychology at the University of Pittsburgh and a practitioner, and was elected president of the Pennsylvania Psychological Association before assuming her position at APA. Dr. Dunivin, who has spent her APA fellowship working for Sen. Daniel Inouye (D–Hawaii), is an independent practitioner and served as president of the Hawaii Psychological Association. Sen. Inouye is the prime congressional sponsor of the PDP.

The three military psychologists selected for the fellowship are Captain Brian Pheiffer and Captain Elaine Rush of the U.S. Air Force and Commander James Parker of the U.S. Navy.

Both civilian psychologists, sworn in last Thursday, will be assigned the rank of major and will begin their first year of the fellowship, along with the military psychologists, at the Uniformed Services University of the Health Sciences (USUHS) in Bethesda, Maryland. The first year will consist of didactic classwork. The second year of training will be a clinical practicum conducted jointly by the Departments of Psychology and Psychiatry at Walter Reed Army Medical Center in Washington. After successful completion of the fellowship, the psychologists will be obligated to serve three years in selected assignments within the Department of Defense.

"The issue of prescription privileges for psychologists and other non-physician providers has been a controversial one within the health care community for the past few years," stated APA's executive director for professional practice, Russ Newman, Ph.D., J.D. "The merit of this program is that it takes the issue out of the arena of polarized rhetoric and places it with an unbiased institution to test the feasibility of expanding prescription privileges beyond medical providers to help fill an unmet public need for services."

The current director of the PDP is Lieutenant Colonel Fred Tamayo, Ph.D., a psychologist with the U.S. Army Medical Service Corps and chief of the Department of Psychology at Walter Reed. The director of training for the PDP is Colonel Marvin Oleshansky, M.D., U.S. Army Medical Corps, a psychiatrist with fellowship training in both psycho-pharmacology and clinical pharmacology. For more information about the fellowship, these directors can be reached at 202/576-1065 or 1066.

---

e. Education and training. Graduate training in psychology typically consists of five years beyond undergraduate training, and it culminates with the award of the doctoral degree. The degree is awarded usually the PhD, but it also may be the PsyD or the EdD. Many psychologists then pursue continuing education, either through lengthy postdoctoral programs or through more time-limited and possibly informal workshops and study groups. Degrees in areas of psychology that are unrelated to practice often follow an apprentice model of science training and there is great variability among them. Degrees in practice areas are more standardized. The most comprehensive account of the nature of this training can be found in the *Criteria for Accreditation of Doctoral Training Programs and Internships in Professional Psychology*, a document developed and published by the American Psychological Association Accreditation office.

Professional training in psychology typically follows the scientist/practitioner model. This approach was initially developed at the Boulder Conference and has been reaffirmed at every major psychological training conference devoted to graduate education. An alternative approach, the practitioner model, also has been developed recently. This model focuses on the development of applied skills, but it does so with a clear accompanying commitment to the scientific knowledge base of psychology.

Professional training in psychology is subject to accreditation by the American Psychological Association. The curriculum of a professional training program in psychology usually requires a minimum of three full-time academic years of resident graduate study. Instruction is provided in scientific and professional ethics and standards, research design and methodology, statistics, psychological measurement, and history of systems of psychology. The student must demonstrate competence in substantive areas that include, but are not limited to:

1. Biological bases of behavior (e.g., physiological psychology, comparative psychology, neuropsychology, sensation, and psychopharmacology);
2. Cognitive–affective bases of behavior (e.g., learning, memory, perception, cognition, thinking, motivation, and emotion);
3. Social bases of behavior (e.g., social psychology; cultural, ethnic, and group processes; sex roles; and organizational and systems theory);
4. Individual behavior (e.g., personality theory, human development, individual differences and abnormal psychology).

In addition to these academic requirements, students also are required to undertake broad based training in particular practice skills related to their areas of study. For the health service provider, training imparts skills such as psychodiagnosis, psychological assessment, and psychological intervention. These techniques are taught in the context of their theoretical and scientific bases, consistent with the status of psychology as a science/profession. Students also receive instruction and supervision in ethical conduct and in the values of professional and scientific responsibility and integrity. The doctoral program concludes with the production of a major scholarly product, usually a doctoral dissertation, in an area relevant to the student's training and interest.

The student in a health service delivery branch of psychology must complete a full year internship. Internships also are subject to accreditation by the American Psychological Association. The internship provides the student with extensive experience in assuming responsibility for professional roles and responsibilities, while also providing careful supervision and role modeling. More advanced training and experience take place with skills such as psychodiagnosis, psychological assessment, and psychological intervention. In this way, the internship prepares the student, upon licensure, to function as an independent professional.

f. Regulation of licensure. The practice of psychology as an autonomous health profession has been regulated by law in each state and in the District of Columbia since 1977. Although regulations differ from state to state, most jurisdictions require a doctoral degree, two years of supervised experience, and an examination procedure in order to award a license to a candidate. The examination recognizes the foundation of the practice of psychology in the science of psychology, and so it includes basic science as well as practice items. Following licensure, commensurate with the role of the independent professional, and consistent with training in the science/profession of psychology, the psychologist must maintain and continuously upgrade skills in service delivery. This is an ethical requirement for all psychologists and a statutory requirement for many psychologists.

As in some other professions, the license in psychology is generic. Because the state does not recognize specialty practice, the profession has the responsibility of determining who, through training and experience, is competent to offer health services. The APA Ethics Code, psychological standards, and many statutory regulations clearly state that licensed psychologists must practice within the areas of their competency. Psychologists who wish to expand their areas of competence may do so through respecialization programs, postdoctoral programs, or continuing education programs.

g. Confidentiality. *Ethics Code 5.02:* Psychologists have a primary obligation and take reasonable precautions to respect the confidentiality rights of those with whom they work or consult, recognizing that confidentiality may be established by law, institutional rules, or professional or scientific relationships.

h. Documentation standards. Psychologists keep documentation concerning all clients. These records not only serve to protect clients' and therapists' rights but also help the psychologist to develop and deliver more effective treatment plans. In addition, these documents can be transferred to other mental health professionals who may treat the client after initial psychological treatment. Documentation kept by psychologists is not only guided by APA guidelines, but also by local and federal laws.

j. Scope of practice. The APA's *General Guidelines for Providers of Psychological Services* includes an explicit definition of the range of services provided by psychologists:

1. Evaluation, diagnosis, and assessment of the functioning of individuals, groups, and organizations.
2. Interventions, preventive and ameliorative, that facilitate the functioning of individuals, groups, and organizations;
3. Consultation relating to 1 and 2;
4. Program development services in the areas of 1, 2, and 3; and
5. Administration and supervision of psychological services.
6. Evaluation of all psychological services.

Psychologists as health care providers offer these services for both mental and general health concerns. They engage in preventive and rehabilitative activities, deliver services in community and private settings, and serve advocacy functions for their patients. They function independently when appropriate, and in multidisciplinary efforts wherever needed. Thus, psychologists are an integral part of a network of health care providers who are available to respond to pressing health and community problems. In addition to these services, psychologists teach at levels ranging from secondary school through postgraduate programs, and they are involved extensively in applied and basic research projects, including the assessment of health delivery services. Psychologists have the ability and the inclination to develop solutions to important community problems and to assess the adequacy of those solutions.

k. Contributions of psychology to MH/SA care. Psychology is a behavioral science that is concerned with how people behave; how they think and feel; and how changes in these behaviors, thoughts, and feelings can be produced. We know that the probability of contracting many illnesses, ranging from the common cold to severe and life-threatening disorders, is increased by stress. We also know that the risk from a majority of the leading causes of death in the United States could be reduced substantially through a change in the behavioral habits of the patient. For example, cancer can be reduced through a decrease in smoking, heart attacks could be reduced through changes in smoking and in diet, many accidents would not occur if not for alcohol abuse, and AIDS often results from unsafe sexual practices. Recent studies of people with a range of illnesses suggest that a greater emphasis on emotional well-being could serve the public health and save the nation money. Psychology has had a significant impact on many aspects of modern life, with health care the fastest growing area of psychological practice. Contributions have come from every specialty area including clinical, neuropsychology, behavioral medicine, and health psychology.

As experts in understanding behavior and in behavior change, psychologists have an important public health role to play in promoting health and reducing disease. The use of psychological interventions, particularly of a brief, focused type, has been demonstrated to improve the health of patients while reducing overall costs of general health care substantially. Psychologists, with their clinical expertise and research based educations, have an important primary role to play in the health care of the citizens of this nation, by treating the ill, preventing disease, and promoting health.

Psychologists have made and will continue to make positive contributions to MH/SA care and health care. These contributions are evident throughout the mental health literature and in the mental health delivery systems throughout the country. Psychologists have made contributions in areas such as primary care, AIDS, violence, multicultural training, disease prevention, and neuroscience. To understand the vast contributions that psychology has made to mental health and health delivery systems one must research the literature on specific topics of interest.

l. Resources

American Psychological Association (1986). *Psychology as a health care profession.* Washington, DC: Author.

American Psychological Association (1992a). Ethical principles of psychologists and code of conduct. *American Psychologist, 47,* 1597–1611.

American Psychological Association (1992b). *Milestones in psychology practice: 1892–1992.* Washington, DC: Author.

American Psychological Association (1993). Record keeping guidelines. *American Psychologist, 48,* 984–986.

American Psychological Association, Board of Professional Affairs, Committee on Professional Standards. (1987). General guidelines for providers of psychological services. *American Psychologist, 47*, 712–723.
American Psychological Association, Committee on Professional Practice and Board of Professional Affairs (1985). *A hospital practice primer for psychologists.* Washington, DC: Author.
Corsini, J. (Ed.). (1984). *Encyclopedia of Psychology: Vol. II.* New York: Wiley.
Striker, G. (1994). *Roles, functions, and contributions of psychologists.* Unpublished manuscript.

2. Nurses[4]

a. Definition. Psychiatric–mental health nursing involves the diagnosis and treatment of human responses to actual or potential mental health problems. Psychiatric–mental health nursing is a specialized area of nursing practice employing theories of human behavior as its science and purposeful use of self as its art. Psychiatric–mental health nurses deliver primary mental health care. Primary mental health care is initiated at the first point of contact with the mental health care system. It includes the continuous and comprehensive services necessary for promotion of optimal mental health, the prevention of mental illness, health maintenance, management, and/or referral of mental and physical health problems, diagnosis and treatment of mental disorders and their sequelae, and rehabilitation. Because of its scope, psychiatric–mental health nursing is necessarily holistic, stressing the needs and strengths of the whole person. Diagnosis of human responses to actual or potential mental health problems involves the application of theory to human phenomena through the processes of assessment, planning, intervention or treatment, and evaluation. Theories providing a basis for psychiatric–mental health nursing practice are derived from various sources, including those from nursing as well as the biological, cultural, environmental, psychological, and sociological sciences.

b. History. There are 2 million nurses licensed in the United States. Of the 204,834 members of American Nurses Association's (ANA) constituent state groups, there are 12,467 who report psychiatric and mental health nursing as their area of practice. During the 1960s, psychiatric–mental health nursing emerged. The focus was on meeting the identified psychosocial needs of general hospital patients. Crisis intervention, brief psychotherapy modalities, and mental health consultation were used by psychiatric nurses. In the 1970s, greater emphasis was placed on prevention and early treatment of emotional problems among nonpsychiatric patients and on mental health consultation to primary care providers.

The impact of the nursing shortage in the United States, with reduced numbers entering the field, has been of concern for a number of years. The effect on psychiatric nursing of decreases in enrollments at the graduate/specialist level has continued in recent years. Psychiatric and mental health nursing became the "trend setter" and provided leadership for nursing in the United States in the 1970s and early 1980s.

c. Nursing practice ethics. Respect for client autonomy, dignity, cultural beliefs, and confidentiality is of particular concern in psychiatric–mental health

---

[4]"Interdisciplinary Approaches: Nursing" was developed by Sarah Stanley, MS, RN, CNA, CS and Sandra Talley, MN, RN, ANP.

nursing. Nurses serve as advocates for the best interests of the client and are accountable to demonstrate a nonjudgmental and nondiscriminatory attitude that is sensitive to client diversity. Issues of vulnerability such as violation of informed consent, abuse of client's rights, unethical behavior, and illegal acts require special vigilance on the part of the nurse who is responsible to protect the client and to report practices that compromise the public's right for humane and appropriate care. Nurses working with psychiatric–mental health clients are prepared to recognize the special nature of the provider-patient relationship and take steps to assure that therapeutic relationships are conducted in a manner that fulfills the responsibilities stipulated in the Code for Nurses.

Standard V of the ANA's (1982) *Standards of Psychiatric and Mental Health Nursing Practice* state that the psychiatric–mental health nurse's decisions and actions on behalf of patients are determined in an ethical manner with the rationale that the public's trust and rights to humane psychiatric–mental health care are upheld by professional nursing practice that puts the best interests of the client first. The foundation of psychiatric–mental health nursing practice is the development of a therapeutic relationship with the client. The psychiatric–mental health nurse engages in therapeutic interactions and relationships which promote and support the healing process. Boundaries need to be established to safeguard the client's well-being and to prevent the development of intimate or sexual relationships.

d. Current developments. The national focus for psychiatric and mental health in the 1990s is on improving service systems at the local level, integrating care, improving service system organization, reaching the consumer, allocating financial resources, resolving legal issues, overcoming stigma, and recognizing nurses as qualified providers. The national research agenda is concentrated on the chronically mentally ill and reaching underserved populations, such as the rural, the poor, and children/adolescents in need of mental health services. Child and adolescent and liaison–consultation psychiatric nursing are areas that are clearly a part of the historical evolution of psychiatric–mental health nursing.

e. Psychiatric rehabilitation. Nursing's involvement in the area of rehabilitation for the chronically mentally ill is carried out in two settings: First in the community or outpatient settings and second in the inpatient, long-term state mental institutions. It is believed that these patients develop pervasive impairments in social, vocational, and adaptive functioning that are often of greater significance than the symptoms of their illness. There may be major impact on the degree of autonomy needed for transition to community life and activities of self-care. Educational and socialization programs have been developed by psychiatric nurses with the goal of producing measurable gains in functioning so that patients would have access to more opportunities for placement, be more successful in the community, and eventually live in the least restrictive environment possible.

f. Education and credentialing

Education. Although there are various educational paths to become a registered nurse (e.g., associate, bachelors, and doctoral level degrees, and programs for non-nurse college graduates), the bachelor's and master's levels of education are considered necessary for developing psychiatric nursing expertise. A "basic" level psychiatric nurse has a bachelor's degree and skills beyond the novice level in caring for persons with psychiatric and/or emotional problems. Master's level preparation provides specialization in psychiatric nursing, and prepares the graduate for independent, consultative, and educational roles in the delivery of mental health care. Master's prepared clinical specialists (the clinical title of advanced practice psychiatric nurses) provide psychotherapy through individual, group, and family modalities; case management; consultation and liaison service within nonpsychiatric settings; and monitoring and/or prescription of psychopharmacological agents.

Educational programs are located in institutions of higher learning within colleges or schools of nursing. Programs must be accredited by the National League for Nursing. Baccalaureate programs usually provide at least one quarter or semester of coursework and clinical experience in psychiatric nursing. Additional emphases in mental health care are integrated in courses in psychology, communication skills, growth and development, and family environments. Master's programs are usually one calendar year or two academic years in length. Coursework and clinical practice are aimed at preparing graduates who can diagnose and treat mental, emotional, and neurobiological problems within the psychiatric specialty. Skills in assessment, differential diagnosis, planning, intervention, and evaluation are developed within standards consistent with the other mental health disciplines of social work, psychology, and psychiatry. As in other disciplines, these therapeutic skills are shaped by the philosophy of nursing. Curriculum projects are a regular part of the planning meetings for the Society for Education and Research in Psychiatric–Mental Health Nursing (SERPN).

Credentialing. The American Nurses Association provides certification examinations for nurses in various specialties. For psychiatric nursing there is one generalist or basic level examination and two advanced clinical specialist examinations (adult and child/adolescent). Certification is available to RN's with associate (until 1998) and bachelor's level education; specialist certification is available to master's prepared nurses who have completed two years of supervised therapy with clients. Renewal of certification occurs every five years with continued clinical practice and continuing education credits in the area.

g. Regulation of licensure

Registered nurse licensure. Registered nurses must be licensed, to practice by a state board of nursing. Requirements for licensure include passage of a national registered nurse examination and demonstration of safe practice. There are 50 states and 3 territorial areas that operate under these guidelines. Further delineation of practice standards, educational requirements, and conduct are found in each state's Nurse Practice Act.

Advanced practice licensure. Additional regulations and/or licensure requirements are found in many states' Nurse Practice Acts. These states have licensed, certified, or otherwise granted advanced practice status (e.g., APRN) to nurses practicing in advanced roles such as nurse practitioner, clinical specialist, and nurse midwife. Advanced licensure is considered necessary to legally expand the practice base (e.g., diagnosis, treatment, and prescriptive practice) of nursing for those with advanced education and prevent those without such training from engaging in activities beyond the scopes of their practice. Requirements for advanced licensure usually include an advanced degree (master's or doctorate) in a specialty area, national certification, and coursework specific to advanced practice activities (e.g., assessment, pharmacology, and psychotherapy). With advanced practice licensure and regulation, other governing boards such as advanced practice peer review committees and prescriptive practice boards have been created to oversee specific practice parameters. These boards regulate the practice activities specific to their purpose and authorize applicants access to the practice privileges.

h. Confidentiality of client and therapist. The practice of nursing does not typically have "client–doctor" or "client–lawyer" confidentiality protection under Nurse Practice Acts. Instead, nurse–client confidentiality is bound by policies or laws regarding the need to report suspected abuse; the "duty to warn" others likely to be harmed by a client being care for by the nurse; and the duty to protect the client from self-harm or from harming others.

Client–nurse confidentiality is further defined according to standards of nursing practice that respect the rights to privacy of individuals under the nurse's care. Information about clients is considered confidential and is not released to others without consent of the client. In another vein, nursing typically strives to provide care within the context of the client's life system, and therefore needs to take into account the care delivered by other providers and the impact of illness and treatment on the client's social system.

i. Documentation standards. Standards of documentation are necessary for communication between parties involved in the delivery of care. Specific detail within psychiatric specialties is related to the domain of care and the common language used between professionals to describe signs, symptoms, diagnoses, treatment plans, and evaluation methodologies. Documentation is also used for reimbursement fees as well as being a legal documentation of the care provided to the client and evaluation of the client's progress and response to treatment. Documentation forms vary between systems of care, companies reimbursing service delivery, and accrediting bodies.

j. Scope of practice. The scope of psychiatric–mental health nursing practice is differentiated according to the level of practice and the role of the nurse. Individual nurses are accountable for identifying their practice parameters within their state nurse practice act, code of ethics, and professional practice standards, and according to their own personal competency to perform particular activities or functions (including psychotherapy and prescriptive practice). The nurse's competence is circumscribed by his or her education, knowledge, experience, and abilities. While psychiatric–mental health nurses are accountable for their own nursing practice, they have a professional responsibility to collaborate and coordinate care with others who may be working with a client and with those whose expertise can enhance the quality of service.

k. Unique contributions of nursing to MH/SA care. Mental health care is provided by the four core mental health disciplines: psychology, social work, psychiatric nursing, and psychiatry. While there are standard, accepted techniques within mental health care, practitioners of each each discipline typically view problems and interventions from their own philosophy developed within their profession. Nursing, like psychiatry, is built on a foundation of generic health care that includes physical interventions and delivery of care to clients during acute episodes of illness. The other domains of nursing practice have been the community and the client's home. These early experiences have important implications for expanding traditional mental health therapies within a nursing framework.

The use of touch with clients receiving mental health care has long been regarded as an intervention likely to be misinterpreted or to cause untoward reactions from the client. Nurses know how to touch clients for procedural interventions such as reading blood pressures, or giving physical examinations and injections. Touch has also been used as a comfort measure or for reassurance when touch is judged appropriate in a situation—that is, when the nurse assesses that the touching will be viewed as a natural extension of the nurse's interaction, and there will not be misinterpretations of the touch as being sexual or aggressive. Determinants of appropriate touching encounters are based on the age of the client and the nurse, the respective genders of each individual, the client's mood and state of health at the moment, and the existing relationship between the two individuals (Tomasini, 1990).

Case management is another technique shaped by nursing's tradition of public health nursing home visiting, and providing care in environments where the client resides. Use of the milieu is a critical component of case management. This may include a residential program, community activities, family relationships, and so forth where there is a need to help clients solve problems within the context of their social milieu.

Specific groups of clients requiring mental health care are those with compromised physical conditions. This includes clients who are frail and elderly, those who are HIV positive or have AIDS, and others with chronic medical conditions requiring complicated health care regimes (e.g., diabetes, TB, hepatitis, and dementia). In these instances nursing brings the familiarity of general health care into psychiatric treatment, improved interaction with health care providers, and oversight of the health care regimen. Improved interaction and careful monitoring of treatment outcomes provide for a more comprehensive treatment plan.

During the past 15 years, approximately 25 states have legalized prescriptive authority privileges for advanced practice psychiatric nurses. Prescriptive authority legislation usually stipulates requirements in the following areas:

- Master's level education;
- Coursework in pharmacology;
- Drug selection limited by formulary or scope of practice; and
- Mechanisms for physician consultation or collaboration.

Advantages of this legislation have been increased access to specialist–practitioners capable of providing pharmacological and psychotherapeutic interventions; reduced cost compared with seeing two separate individuals (one for therapy and the other for psychopharmacological); and improved care for clients who received medication management from a nonspecialty system of care.

I. Resources

Abraham, I. L. (1992). Integrating the bio into the biopsychological: Understanding and treating biological phenomena in psychiatric-mental health nursing. *Archives of Psychiatric Nursing, 6* (5), 296–305.

American Nurses Association. (1976). *Statement on psychiatric and mental health nursing practice.* Kansas City, MO: Author.

American Nurses Association. (1980). *Nursing: A social policy statement.* Kansas City, MO: Author.

American Nurses Association. (1982). *Standards of psychiatric and mental health nursing practice.* Kansas City, MO: Author

American Nurses Association. (1985). *ANA code for nurses with interpretive statements.* Kansas City, MO: Author.

American Nurses Association. (1985). *Standards of child and adolescent psychiatric and mental health nursing practice.* Kansas City, MO: Author.

American Nurses Association. (1986). *Psychiatric and mental health clinical nurse specialists: distribution and utilization.* Kansas City, MO: Author.

American Nurses Association. (1990). *Standards of psychiatric consultation–liaison nursing practice.* Kansas City, MO: Author.

American Nurses Association. (1991). *Nursing's agenda for health care reform.* Kansas City, MO: Author.

American Nurses Association. (1993). *Health care reform: Essential mental health services.* Washington, DC: Author.

Bachrach, L. (1993). Continuity of care and approaches to case management for long-term mentally ill patients. *Hospital and Community Psychiatry, 44,* 465–468.

Boyd, M. A., Morris, M. M., & Little, J. (1991). An educational inpatient rehabilitation program. *Journal of Psychosocial Nursing, 29* (1), 24.

Chamberlain, J. (1987). Update on psychiatric-mental health nursing education at the federal level. *Archives of Psychiatric Nursing, 1* (2), 132.

Collins-Colon, T. (1990). Do it yourself: Medication management for community based clients. *Journal of Psychosocial Nursing, 28* (6), 25.

Connolly, P. M. (1991). Services for the underserved: A nurse-managed center for the chronic mentally ill. *Journal of Psychosocial Nursing, 29* (1),

Fox, J. (1986). *Essential and critical knowledge for psychiatric–mental health nursing in the twenty-first century.* NIMH Publication 56–57.

Fox, J. (1991). Psychiatric nursing: Directions for the future. In Aiken & C. Fagin, *Nursing and health policy issues in the 1990s.*

Fox, J. M., Merwin, E. L., et al. (1990). Human resources. In R. W. Manderscheid & M. A. Sonnenschein (Eds.), *Mental health, United States, 1990.* Washington, DC: United States Government Printing Office.

Henderson, V., & Nite, G. (1978). *Principles and practice of nursing.* New York: MacMillan.

Institute of Medicine. (1989). *Research on children and adolescents with mental, behavioral & developmental disorders.* (Pub IOM-89-07). Washington, DC: National Academy Press.

Jones, S. L., & Jones, P. K. (1987). Research in psychiatric and mental health nursing: The emergence of scientific rigor. *Archives of Psychiatric Nursing, 1* (3), 155.

Krauss J. (1987). Nursing, madness and mental health. *Archives of Psychiatric Nursing, 1,* 3–15.

Krauss J. (1993). *Health care reform: Essential mental health services.* Washington, DC: American Nurses Association.

Liaschenko, J. (1989). Changing paradigms within psychiatry: Implications for nursing research. *Archives of Psychiatric Nursing, 111* (3), 153–158.

McBride, A. B. (1987). Developing a women's mental health research agenda. *Image, 19* (1), 4–8.

McBride, A. B. (1990). Psychiatric nursing in the 1990s. *Archives of Psychiatric Nursing, 4* (1), 21–28.

McBride, A. B., & Friedenburg, E. C. (1989). Research opportunities at the National Institute of Mental Health. *Image, 21* (4), 251–253.

Michaels, C. (1992). Carondelet St. Mary's nursing enterprise. *Nursing Clinics of North America, 27,* 77–85.
Mound, B., Gylulay, R., Khan, P., & Goering, P. (1991). The expanded role of nurse case managers. *Journal of Psychosocial Nursing, 28* (7), 7–12.
Murphy, S., & Hoeffer, B. (1987). The evolution of subspecialties in psychiatric and mental health nursing. *Archives of Psychiatric Nursing, 1* (3), 145–154.
National Institute of Mental Health. (1987). *Psychiatric-mental health nursing: Educational blueprint in the 21st century.* Washington, DC: U.S. Department of Health and Human Services.
O'Toole, A., & Loomis, M. (1989). Classifying human responses in psychiatric–mental health nursing. In *Classification systems for describing nursing practice: Working papers.* Kansas City, MO: American Nurses Association.
Peplau, H. (1980). The psychiatric nurse-accountable? To whom? For what? *Perspectives in Psychiatric Care, 128.*
Peplau, H. (1982). Some reflections on earlier days in psychiatric nursing. *Journal of Psychiatric and Mental Health Services, 20* (8), 17–24.
Pothier, P. (1987). The future of psychiatric nursing—revisited. *Archives of Psychiatric Nursing, 1* (5), 299–300
Pothier, P., Stuart, G., Puskar, K., & Babich, K. (1990). Dilemmas and directions for psychiatric nursing in the 1990s. *Archives of Psychiatric Nursing, 4* (5), 284–291.
Ricci, M. S. (1990). The new after-care clinic: Treating individuals rather than masses. *Journal of Psychosocial Nursing, 28* (8), 18.
Stanley, S. (1990). Review of the institute of medicine report on children and adolescents. *Journal of Child & Adolescent Psychiatric Mental Health Nursing, 3* (2), 62.
Talley, S. L. (1992). Prescriptive authority for psychiatric clinical specialists: Framing the issues. *Archives of Psychiatric Nursing, 4* (2), 71–82.
Tomasini, N. (1990). The use of touch with the hospitalized psychiatric patient. *Archives of Psychiatric Nursing, 4,* 213–220.
VanDongen, C. J., & Jambunthan, J. (1992). Pilot study results: The psychiatric RN case manager. *Journal of Psychosocial Nursing, 30* (11), 11–14.
Whall, A. (1986). *The phenomena of concern to psychiatric–mental health nursing practice: Implications for the 21st century.* NIMH Publication 45–55.
Worley, N. (1990). Improving the physical health-mental health interface for the chronically mentally ill. Could nurse case managers make a difference? *Archives of Psychiatric Nursing, 4,* 108–113.

3. *Social Workers*

a. Definition. The National Association of Social Workers (NASW) defines social work as "the professional activity of helping individuals, groups, or communities enhance or restore their capacity for social functioning and creating societal conditions favorable to this goal. Social work practice consists of the professional application of social work values, principles, and techniques to one or more of the following ends: helping people obtain tangible services, providing counseling and psychotherapy with individuals, families, and groups; helping communities or groups provide or improve social and health services; and participating in relevant legislative processes. The practice of social work requires knowledge of human development and behavior; of social, economic, and cultural institutions; and of the interactions of all these factors" (*Standards for Social Service Manpower,* 1973, pp. 4–5).

b. History. Enormous changes have taken place in mental health practice in America in the last three centuries. The European experience as well as homegrown reform movements have all had an impact on the treatment of persons with mental health problems. In colonial times, policies were nonexistent. During the nineteenth and first half of the twentieth centuries the emphasis was on institutionalization. States and later the federal government assumed responsibility for the mental health care of their citizens. Deinstitutionalization has been public policy since the late 1950s. Today the state systems, the private sector, and hospitals are components of a system that focuses on community mental health.

The social work profession developed within this changing historical context. Many of the participants in the nineteenth century reform movements were prototypes of today's social workers. Pioneer mental health social workers carved out a niche for themselves during the emergence of the social work profession in the early twentieth century.

Several social workers held positions in hospitals for the psychiatrically impaired in the first decade of the twentieth century. Initially they assumed the responsibility for making linkages with the community. In 1906, the first trained social worker was hired as an aftercare agent to help patients find housing, employment, and other resources in the community. Mary C. Jarrett, a caseworker who became the Chief of Social Service of the Boston Psychopathic Hospital, coined the term *psychiatric social work* and pioneered the field's development. In 1918, the first training program for psychiatric social workers was sponsored by the Boston Psychopathic Hospital, the National Committee for Mental Hygiene, and Smith College. Around the same time other schools of social work began to include psychiatric studies in their educational programs. The 1930s and 1940s saw the expansion of outpatient services and the development of mental health service delivery teams consisting of a psychiatrist, a psychologist, and a social worker.

By the late 1930s, psychiatric social workers had established themselves in the Red Cross and Veterans' Administration services, public and private hospitals, child guidance clinics, mental hygiene clinics and societies, general hospital clinics, educational institutions, state departments of mental hygiene, public health nursing organizations, family welfare agencies, and private practice. Their functions varied by the setting. The ability to penetrate the community's system of services was the distinguishing feature of the social worker employed in mental health settings.

A professional membership association was founded in 1926 for psychiatric social workers specializing in clinical work with mentally ill people or working in mental health settings. It merged with six other social work membership organizations in 1955 to form the National Association of Social Workers (NASW).

Two world wars, the establishment of the National Institute of Mental Health, President Kennedy's "bold new approach," and President's Reagan's Omnibus Budget Reconciliation Act have affected the climate and way in which clinical social work in community mental health has been practiced. The current health care debate of the 1990s will also have an impact.

c. **Social work ethics.** Social workers currently subscribe to the NASW Code of Ethics as adopted by the Delegate Assembly of NASW in 1979 (effective 1980) and amended at the 1990 and 1993 NASW Delegate Assemblies. The principles contained in the code are both prescriptive and proscriptive. They represent the ideas and convictions of social work practitioners and scholars about the obligations of the contemporary social worker. The Code of Ethics includes principles that relate to the social worker's (a) conduct and comportment, (b) ethical responsibility to clients, (c) ethical responsibility to colleagues, (d) ethical responsibility to employer and employing organizations, (e) ethical responsibility to the social work profession, and (f) ethical responsibility to society. Values and ethical issues will continually permeate the profession and examination of these issues will continue. See Reamer (1990) for discussion of the code.

d. Current developments. These changes include a renewed focus on the biological factors as primary in the etiology of mental illness, the introduction of and controversies surrounding revised editions of the American Psychiatric Association's *Diagnostic and Statistical Manual of Mental Disorders*, a recognition that severely mentally disabled people who live in the community are in great need of services, and the emergence of new client and consumer groups.

Research is documenting the effectiveness of medication in allowing many people with serious mental and emotional illnesses to live normal or near normal lives. Because, psychotropic medications have become an important intervention for use with individuals at all stages of life, social workers must be knowledgeable about psychopharmacology.

The lack of community resources for the deinstitutionalized and the need to find an effective balance between private and government efforts represent some difficult problems facing the field. Innovative approaches, including community services for people with chronic mental illness, will require learning new roles and expanding the expectations of client's abilities. The field is changing and expanding and offers social workers a chance to participate in these changes in a meaningful and positive way.

e. Psychiatric social work. *Clinical social work practice* is the current term for psychiatric social work that occurs in a mental health setting. The psychiatric social worker provides psychotherapy and other social services for those with mental disorders and, in collaboration with the psychiatrist and other members of the mental health team, works with patients' family members. The worker usually has a MSW or higher degree and additional experience in working with psychiatric problems. Because the social work professional is emphasizing the common elements of his or her various specialties, psychiatric social work is not so distinct as it formerly was.

f. Education and credentialing

Education. Social work education in the United States traces its roots to 1898 when the New York Charity Organization Society offered a summer training course for charity workers. During the next two decades, social work education became more formal and systematic. By 1919, 17 schools of social work in the United States and Canada organized the Association of Training Schools for Professional Social Work. The association soon changed its name to the American Association of Schools of Social Work (AASSW) and, by 1927, developed educational standards that were required for membership in the organization. These standards quickly evolved into a set of academic and organizational requirements designed to ensure that students were adequately prepared for professional practice. By 1935, these standards required that schools of social work be affiliated with universities and, by 1939, only schools offering two years of graduate study were eligible for membership (Kendall, 1991).

In 1942, dissatisfied with the AASSW requirement that social work eduction be offered exclusively at the graduate level and interested in preparing undergraduate students for public welfare practice, several baccalaureate programs established the National Association of Schools of Social Administration (NASSA). NASSA members were land-grant colleges, private schools, and state universities offering a baccalaureate social work degree and, in a few cases, an additional year leading to the master's degree. In 1943, NASSA was recognized as the official accrediting body for baccalaureate programs.

The existence of two national accrediting organizations purporting to represent social work education was confusing and problematic for students, educators, practitioners, employers, and the public. As a result, in 1946, a coordinating group known as the National Council on Social Work Education (NCSWE) was established to work out a solution. NCSWE consisted of representatives from 13 professional social work associations and governmental and voluntary agencies. Supported by a grant from the Carnegie Foundation, NCSWE conducted a comprehensive study of social work education. The report, written by Ernest Hollis and Alice Taylor (1951), recommended that the professions come together to develop and support a single organization that would be responsible for educational and accreditation policies and procedures. The collaborative work of the NCSWE and the Hollis–Taylor report led, in 1952, to the creation of the Council on Social Work Education (CSWE) as the successor to AASSW and NASSA.

CSWE was given the responsibility for setting standards for social work education and accrediting master's degree programs. Baccalaureate programs were viewed by CSWE as preprofessional at that time and were not offered accreditation. "A first step in the direction of standards for baccalaureate programs was taken in 1962 when criteria were developed to govern the admission of undergraduate social work departments to *constituent membership* in CSWE" (Kendall, 1991). In 1967, additional criteria were developed, including one on preparing students for beginning practice. Three years later, CSWE issued new criteria and began a system of official approval of baccalaureate programs. In 1974, accreditation was made available to baccalaureate programs.

In conformance with the requirements of the Council on Postsecondary Accreditation (COPA) and the U.S. Department of Education, the Commission on Accreditation of the Council on Social Work Education is responsible for formulating the standards, policies, and procedures for accrediting baccalaureate and master's programs of social work education and proposing them to CSWE's Board of Directors for adoption. CSWE's Commission on Educational Policy is responsible for developing the Curriculum Policy Statement. After adoption by CSWE's Board of Directors, the Curriculum Policy Statement becomes the official policy governing curricula offered at the baccalaureate and master's levels and functions as the basis for the accreditation standards used to evaluate social work education programs. CSWE periodically revises its Curriculum Policy Statement and its accrediting standards.

Doctoral education in social work is a late twentieth-century development. The number of doctoral programs grew slowly in the first half century, but there have been dramatic increases in the 1960s and again in the 1980s. Despite this dramatic program growth, the total number of doctoral graduates has remained nearly constant throughout the last decade. The Group for the Advancement of Doctoral Education (GADE) was founded almost 20 years ago by leading faculty in schools of social work concerned about the pressures facing their doctoral programs. GADE provides a forum for sharing ideas and strategies and for strengthening members' efforts at enhancing doctoral education. Social work doctoral programs in accredited universities are controlled by those institutions. The educational program is developed within the philosophy of the host institution.

Credentialing. NASW has led the way in setting standards for professional practice since 1955 with the establishment of the Code of Ethics. All NASW members and credential holders agree to uphold these ethics in social work practice. NASW assures quality social work practice with its professional standards in a wide range of areas including schools, health care settings, long-term care facilities, clinical social work, child protection, mediation, and case management.

In 1962, the Academy of Certified Social Workers (ACSW) was founded by NASW as a separate corporation to establish quality assurance standards and to prepare for the eventual development of a certification system. In 1992, ACSW celebrated its 30th birthday, with 65,000 members certified for independent, self-regulated practice, and it remains the most widely recognized and respected social work credentialing body today. Certification is awarded upon successful completion of a master's degree program, two years of supervision by an ACSW member, and competence on a test of quantative standards.

NASW established a Competence Certification Commission (CCC) to create and maintain credentials that meet the needs of most social workers and that advance the profession. Social work credentials are not mandatory, but social workers wishing to demonstrate their knowledge and experience beyond the basic requirements seek them voluntarily. It helps social workers stay competitive, strengthens consumer confidence in the services provided, promotes a positive image of the profession, and enhances the prestige of social workers among colleagues and other professionals.

The NASW register of clinical social workers, first published in 1976, includes qualified clinical social workers and diplomates in clinical social work. The diplomate in clinical social work was created in 1986 to distinguish advanced clinical practice expertise and is NASW's highest-level professional credential.

In 1991, NASW created the Academy of Certified Baccalaureate Social Workers (ACBSW) credential to give BSWs national professional recognition. The ACBSW requires at least two years of post-BSW supervised social work experience in an agency or organizational setting. The ACBSW credential identified the holder as a social worker who has voluntarily met enduring, uniformly high national standards for practice and who maintains a high level of professional conduct.

In 1992, NASW created the School Social Work Specialist credential for social work practitioners who work in public schools, private schools, preschools, and special education and residential school settings.

g. Regulation of licensure. The NASW has very successfully promoted state licensing (or registration) requirements to assure the public that social work practitioners meet high standards of competence.

Through licensing, social workers are granted a formal governmental authorization to do something that cannot be done legally without that authorization. Although standards vary, most states require practicing social workers to be licensed, certified, or registered. State regulatory boards or the American Association of State Social Work Boards provides information on the different standards and requirements.

h. Confidentiality of client and social worker. Social workers assume that information shared by clients should be kept confidential, but on occasion practitioners need to consider disclosing confidential information. The NASW Code of Ethics states that social workers may reveal confidential information for "compelling professional reasons" but there is no consensus on what conditions warrant such disclosure. In some states, clients have the right of privileged communication that provides grounds for social workers to refuse to disclose information shared by a client to, for example, a court of law. Even in those instances, social workers must sometimes choose between a court order and the client's right to confidentiality.

i. Documentation standards. Case records provide an ongoing picture of the nature of social work involvement with a client, progress in achieving social work goals, and the eventual outcome of the interaction between social worker and client or agency. The type of recording depends on the agency's requirements.

j. Scope of practice. Social work services in mental health are provided by master's degree graduates from accredited schools of social work and social work assistants who hold bachelor's degrees from accredited schools of social work. Social work staff at all levels are licensed or certified following state licensing regulations. Social workers provide services to patients and their families—as members of interdisciplinary teams—by contributing to program development, treatment planning, and review for all patients, and collaborating in the development and maintenance of the therapeutic milieu.

Social workers have particular competence in two areas relevant to mental health services. First, they have a solid working knowledge of community resources and are trained in referring clients for specific services and monitoring the results. Secondly, they specialize in assessing the family and community contexts of mental illness that enable them to make recommendations regarding needed environmental changes.

k. Unique contributions of social work to MH/SA care. Many of the problems dealt with by social workers have traditionally been seen as mental health problems. When behavioral problems are defined as having organic or intrapsychic causes, the mental health system is usually the provider of services. Services are provided either in the public or private sector by psychiatrists, psychologists, social workers, and nurses. It has been estimated that half the professionals who provide mental health services in the United States today are social workers (Zastrow, 1993).

Social workers provide a variety of preventive, diagnostic, and treatment services. Over the years the treatment emphasis has moved from treating the individual to treating the family. Social workers, psychologists, psychiatrists, and psychiatric nurses now work with individuals, families, and groups.

Social workers carry out many different roles within the mental health system. They operate as case managers. They are in aftercare and community support programs for those discharged from mental institutions. They often combine the case manager role with advocating for clients' rights. They carry out roles in planning, administration, and supervision, and help formulate policies and plan programs, especially for those who have been deinstitutionalized. They advocate for legislation and program changes to ensure client rights and to improve services. They also supervise other workers, administer programs, and head agencies.

l. Resources:

Barker, R. L. (1991). *The social work dictionary* (2nd ed.). Washington, DC: NASW Press.

Commission on Accreditation. (1988 & 1991). *Handbook of accreditation standards and procedures.* Alexandria, VA: CSWE.

Group for the Advancement of Doctoral Education (GADE). (1992). *Guidelines for quality in social work doctoral programs* (NIMH Contract No. 278-88-0024).

Hollis, E. V., & Taylor, A. L. (1951). *Social work education in the United States: The report of a study made for the National Council on Social Work Education.* New York: Columbia University Press.

Kendall, K. A. (1991). *The Council on Social Work Education: A history 1952–1988.* Unpublished manuscript.

Libassi, M. F. (1990). *Psychopharmacology in social work education* (NIMH Contract Report). Alexandria, VA: Council on Social Work Education.

Mehr, J. (1992). *Human services concepts and intervention strategies* (5th ed.). Boston: Allyn and Bacon.

Popple, P. R., & Leighninger, L. (1993). *Social work, social welfare, and American society.* Boston: Allyn and Bacon.

Reamer, F. G. (1990). *Ethical dilemmas in social service—A guide for social workers* (2nd ed.). New York: Columbia University Press.

Standards for social service manpower. (1973). Washington, DC: National Association of Social Workers.

Zastrow, C. (1993). *Introduction to social work and social welfare* (5th ed.). California: Brooks/Cole.

4. Other Providers

In addition to psychologists, nurses, and social workers, there are a wide variety of other health and social service providers that the three professions addressed by this curriculum must relate to in rural areas. In assessing community needs, identifying community resources, and developing approaches to community problems, all other providers should be taken into account. In all rural settings, family physicians and other primary care medical personnel must be included in interdisciplinary planning. To the extent that they are present in a particular rural area, pharmacists, licensed counselors, and addiction counselors should also be included. In some rural areas, nonlicensed counselors (e.g., clergy and native healers) have a major role and should be included.

E. Rural Social Service Systems

Although social services are similar throughout the United States, there are some special issues associated with social services organization and delivery in rural areas. For example, a metropolitan area may have a number of offices for each of the social services programs, including community mental health. For rural areas, however, the specific rural community may only be part of a larger regional catchment area. Clients may have to travel to distant locations for services or wait for periodic visits from professionals to the community.

In some cases, formal, funded services may exist. Some services may be provided by volunteers or by agencies such as churches and law enforcement bodies that are not normally considered part of the service delivery system. Therefore, those who work in rural areas must develop specialized skills in knowing how services are—or might be—delivered to clients in rural communities.

Goals

1. Learn to identify key elements of social service systems in rural areas.
2. Understand the process for describing or mapping social service systems.
3. Recognize the points of access to services and their limitations.
4. Understand the linkages and relationships within social service systems.
5. Identify the cultural perspective on use of social services in the community.

Resources

Balacki, M. F. (1988). Assessing the mental health needs in the rural community: A critique of assessment approaches. *Issues in Mental Health Nursing, 9,* 299–315.

Ballew, J. R. (1985). Role of natural helpers in preventing child abuse and neglect. *Social Work, 30,* 37–41.

Bicknell, E. H. (1991). A rural community-based model for care delivery to chronically mentally ill elderly. In A. Bushy (Ed.), *Rural nursing: Vol. II.* Newbury Park, CA: Sage.

Boyer, P. A., & Elkin, B. (guest Eds.). (1989). Rural chronically mentally ill [Special Issue]. *Human Services in the Rural Environment, 12* (4).

Brantly, D., & West, S. (1980). The rural developmentally disabled in an underserved population. *Human Services in the Rural Environment, 5* (2), 17–24.

Cassidy, T. M., Gordon, M. S., & Heller, A. (1981). *The mountains and valleys are mine: A symposium on rural mental health.* Ridgewood, NY: Bren-Tru Press.

Conway-Welch, C. (1991). Issues surrounding the distribution and utilization of nurse nonphysician providers in rural America. *The Journal of Rural Health, 7* (4), supplement.

Coward, R. T. (1987). Factors associated with the configuration of the helping networks of noninstitutionalized elders. *Gerontological Social Work With Families, 10,* 113–132.

Flaskerud, J. H., & Kviz, F. J. (1982). Resources rural consumers indicate they would use for mental health problems. *Community Mental Health Journal, 34,* 229–233.

Horwitz, A. (1978). Family, kin, and friend networks in psychiatric help-seeking. *Social Science and Medicine, 12,* 297–304.

York, R. D., Denton, R. T., & Moran, J. R. (1994). Rural and urban social work practice: Is there a difference? In L. Ginsberg (Ed.), *Social work in rural communities.* Alexandria, VA: Council on Social Work Education.

F. Rural Health, Mental Health, and Substance Abuse Service Systems

All health services in rural communities pose special issues and they extend to mental health and substance abuse services. Summer (1991) states,

> Often the population base in rural areas is simply not large enough to support the type of medical facilities and practitioners available to residents of more densely populated areas. In an emergency, the lack of proximity to care can be life threatening. For routine services, the need to travel great distances can be a deterrent to seeking care. (p. 3)

There are issues involved in arranging care in rural areas that go beyond those of simply finding reimbursement sources. In many cases there is no *infrastructure* for providing services; that is, there are no nearby, available service providers. There is no public transportation that can reasonably be used to reach the service providers. To complicate matters, there are also serious problems of stigma associated, in particular, with rural substance abuse and mental health problems. Confidentiality is potentially difficult to maintain, especially during the process of locating services and finding access to those services.

On the issue of reimbursement or eligibility for services, the same problems remain. The agency that approves providers for Medicaid, for example, may not have a nearby, local office. That may mean the client needs to travel to a distant city in order to obtain eligibility—before any services are received. In general, arranging services for disadvantaged people who need health, mental health, or substance abuse services requires aggressive and imaginative efforts on the part of service providers.

Goals

1. Learn to identify health and MH/SA services in rural communities.
2. Understand the traditional and nontraditional service infrastructure in rural communities.
3. Understand the process for describing the MH/SA service systems (existing providers), their qualifications, and regulatory framework for service delivery.
4. Identify the points of access to services and their limitations.
5. Understand the linkages and relationships between the mental health and health care service system.
6. Recognize the implications of funding mechanisms on funding and providing services.

Resources

Bigbee, J. L. (1992). Frontier areas: Opportunities for NPs' primary care services. *Nurse Practitioner, 17* (9), 47–57.

Flaskerud, J. H., & Kviz, F. J. (1983). Rural attitudes towards and knowledge of mental illness and treatment services. *Community Mental Health Journal, 43,* 229–233.
Flaskerud, J. H., & Kviz, F. J. (1984). Determining the need for mental health services in rural areas. *American Journal of Community Psychology, 12* (4), 497–510.
Holmberg, S. (1988). Physical health problems of the psychiatric client. *Journal of Psychosocial Nursing, 26* (5), 35–39.
Nettekoven, L., & Sunberg, N. (1985). Community assessment methods in rural mental health promotion. *Journal of Rural Community Psychology, 6* (2), 21–43.
Rowley, B. D., and Baldwin, D. C. (1984). Assessing rural community resources for health care: The use of health services catchment area economic marketing studies. *Social Science Medicine, 6,* 525–529.
Stratton, T. D., Gibbons, B., Dunkin, J. W., & Juhl, N. (1993). How states respond to the rural nursing shortage. *Nursing and Health Care, 14* (5), 238–243.
Stratton, T. D., Sudlke, R. L., & Juhl, N. (1993, July). A demographic analysis of nurse shortage counties: Implications for rural nursing policy. University of North Dakota Rural Health Research Center, Office of Rural Health Policy, Grant No. CSR 0000005-01-0.
Summer, L. (1991). *Limited access: Health care for the rural poor* [executive summary]. Washington, DC: Center on Budget and Policy Priorities.
Turner, S. L. (1979). Disability among schizophrenics in a rural community: Services and social support. *Research in Nursing and Health, 2,* 151–161.
Worley, N. K., & Lowery, R. J. (1991). Linkages between community mental health centers and public mental hospitals. *Nursing Research, 40* (5), 298–302.

G. Community Paradigms and Preventive Strategies

Goals

1. Learn the skills associated with organizing the community for solving mental health problems.
2. Identify the skills necessary for successful program design and development.

Helping overcome mental health problems requires attention not only to the individuals and families who experience those problems, but also to the larger system—the community—which can play an important role in preventing, educating about, and helping organize treatment for mental illness. The objective of this unit is to help the trainees become knowledgeable about and able to intervene at the community level.

The pervasive concept is that mental health problems cannot all be solved on a one-to-one basis; problems must also be addressed through community change. One of the outcomes of such *macro work* is the development and design of programs that incorporate new and different approaches to problem-solving in the mental health arena.

There are many skills associated with organizing the community for solving mental health problems. The fundamentals are to help the community identify its problems and needs; rank or prioritize those problems or needs; develop the desire to work on those problems or needs; marshall the resources for resolving them; and implement the solutions chosen by the community.

Program design and development also require a number of skills. Essentially, there are administrative skills that are part of the ability of the professional manager, including the community mental health manager. The skills require setting objectives, developing plans, implementing plans, and evaluating the results.

Resources

Edwards, R. L., & Yankey, J. A. (Eds.). (1989). *Skills for effective human services management.* Washington, DC: NASW Press.

Keys, P. R., & Ginsberg, L. (1987). *New management in human services.* Washington, DC: NASW Press.

Minahan, A. (Ed.). (1987). *Encyclopedia of social work* (18th ed.). Silver Spring, MD: NASW Press.

Parker, M., Quinn, J., Viehl, M., McKinley, A., Polich, C. L., Detzner, D. F., Hartwell, S., & Korn, K. (1992). Case management in rural areas: Definition, clients, financing, staffing, and service delivery issues. In A. Bushy (Ed.), *Rural nursing: Vol. II* (pp. 29–40). Newbury Park, CA: Sage.

Preston, D. B., Young, E., & Koch, P. (1991). AIDS: A perspective from rural counties in Pennsylvania and New York. In A. Bushey (Ed.), *Rural Nursing: Vol. II.* Newbury Park, CA: Sage.

Statewide Office of Rural Health, Washington State & Washington Rural Health Association (1994). *Implementing health care reform: Setting a course for rural Washington.* Seattle, WA: WAMI Rural Health Center.

Stratton, T. D., Gibbons, B., Dunkin, J. W., & Juhl, N. (1993). How states respond to the rural nursing shortage. *Nursing & Health Care, 14* (5), 238–243.

Stratton, T. D., Sudlke, R. L., Juhl, N., Dunkin, J. W., & Geller, J. M. (1993, July). *A demographic analysis of nurse shortage counties: Implications for rural nursing policy.* University of North Dakota Rural Health Research Center, Office of Rural Health Policy, Grant No. CSR-0000005-01-0.

Turner, S. L. (1979). Disability among schizophrenics in a rural community: Services and social support. *Research in Nursing Health, 2,* 151–161.

Worley, N. K., & Lowery, R. J. (1991). Linkages between community mental health centers and public mental hospitals. *Nursing Research, 40* (5), 298–302.

H. Interdisciplinary Team Building

Goals

1. Recognize that the purpose of team building is to provide more efficient and effective care services.
2. Apply group process theories and principles to rural mental health interdisciplinary team building.
3. Understand methods for establishing structure of effective interdisciplinary teams.
4. Be aware of the impact of team members' varying knowledge, competence, and authority issues on team functioning.
5. Define areas of overlapping competency and practice.
6. Recognize barriers to effective collaboration and methods to overcome these barriers.

The interdisciplinary team approach to the delivery of health services to rural areas was studied and a curriculum was developed by the University of Colorado Health Sciences Center (UCHSC) Interdisciplinary Rural Team Training Project. This portion of the curriculum is an adaptation of the work of the UCHSC project to fit the need for MH/SA services in rural areas. Full credit is acknowledged for this valuable material.

In an interdisciplinary team clinical approach, care is integrated and team members actively coordinate care across disciplines and collaborate on patient care decisions. There is an organized distribution of clinical responsibility for a patient's MH/SA problem(s) with each member contributing his or her skills and expertise as indicated. The mix and outcome of the services are regularly evaluated. Open lines of communication must be maintained among the disciplines that integrate diagnosis and treatment as well as individual, family, and community concerns. The team members have joint responsibility for discussions regarding provisions of care for each patient. Team members must be trained in the use of the teamwork concept and tools.

The essential attributes of team members include open-mindedness, tolerance of different perspectives, willingness to experience new modes of interaction, and acceptance of change. When an interdisciplinary team is fully developed, the disciplines understand each other's roles and how to successfully interact, and each individual's personal expectations are explored and either met or modified to achieve team success. A fully integrated team should be egalitarian with each member respecting the role of others. Leadership varies with the specifics of the task(s) and there is recognition that the team contribution is of grater value than the contribution of one member. A truly interdisciplinary, egalitarian team benefits all involved. Providers, teachers, students, and patients all gain tangible advantages, both through improved outcomes of care and a more productive process of care.

Barriers

Within each profession, there are historical factors that make team approaches to practice appear less desirable than individual approaches. Clinicians have been less interested in interacting with each other and more interested in focusing on their own clinical decisions. There are many examples of failed team structures, largely due to poor training, design, and administration of teams. Professional education programs are typically discipline-specific and often do not encourage cross-disciplinary responsibility.

Traditional models of practice and team approaches to practice differ in important ways and evoke quite different responses from the various professions. Traditional models of care are perceived as dividing the body and its treatment into component parts. They are perceived as being at odds with the holistic approach, which requires an interplay of mind, spirit, body and environment and is central to some disciplines. Team members may have different outcome goals that result from their differing values. In addition, common goals and philosophies often are not clearly identified. Differing explanations of patients, team participants, other health care personnel, or administrators can lead to conflict.

The theoretical basis for an interdisciplinary approach is not often taught or modeled in professional education programs. In some areas, there is no common interdisciplinary vocabulary. Professional recognition tends to accrue only within one's own field. The important processes of socialization to the norms of one's own profession tend to occur in isolation from other disciplines. *Disciplinary centrism,* viewing one's own discipline as superior and more relevant, is at least as common in education as in practice. Each discipline's philosophy emphasizes different types of information for clinical problem-solving.

Benefits

For patients

- delivers optimum comprehensive health care by using the expertise of many professions
- provides the most appropriate management for more complex cases
- provides case management addressing complex needs
- integrates group knowledge and activity into an outcome greater than the sum of the contribution of each individual and discipline
- provides collaboration, cooperation, and knowledge-sharing among disciplines
- increases overall quality of life for patient and family
- increases quality of care
- increases cost-effectiveness of care

For providers

- increases personal satisfaction with practice and reduces work-related frustrations, through:

    1. continuous cooperative effort by a stable group of professionals that defines its own tasks and evaluates its own efforts;
    2. greater professional satisfaction from working in a stable situation in which members are supported by the whole team and are assigned tasks appropriate for their training;
    3. a clearer and more consistent relationship between a patient's health status and the care received;
    4. exposure to broader clinical and social issues relevant to a patient's care; and
    5. more efficient and effective administrative decision-making.

- develops communication and negotiation skills to achieve common goals
- rewards communications and interpersonal connection
- promotes collaborative decision-making
- encourages agreement on plans of care
- leads to support of each other
- draws those with parallel patient-care responsibilities into collaborative and educational relationships
- facilitates awareness of alternative decision-making strategies and ethical issues

For faculty

- blends teaching and educational paradigms from different disciplines
- expands appreciation of knowledge and skills of colleagues
- utilizes all available knowledge and resources
- challenges norms and values of each discipline, encouraging improvement and expansion
- provides fun, exhilaration, support, and opportunities for creativity

For students

- provides a broader, more sophisticated education
- promotes participation
- encourages appreciation of contributions of other disciplines
- utilizes broader base of available knowledge and resources
- models strategies for use in future practice
- provides fun, exhilaration, support, and opportunities for creativity

For the MH/SA delivery system

- maximizes the use of available resources and facilities

Resources

DeLeon, P. H., Kjervik, D. K., Kraut, A. G., & VandenBos, G. R. (1985). Psychology and nursing: A natural alliance. *American Psychologist, 40,* 1153–1164.

Drotar, D. (1993). Influences on collaborative activities among psychologists and pediatricians: Implications for practice, training, and research. *Journal of Pediatric Psychology, 18,* 159–172.

Fennell, M., & Sandefur, G. D. (1983). Structural clarity of interdisciplinary teams: A research note. *The Journal of Applied Behavioral Science, 19,* 193–202.

Koeske, G. F., Koeske, R. D., & Mallinger, J. (1993). Perceptions of professional competence: Cross-disciplinary ratings of psychologists, social workers, and psychiatrists. *American Journal of Orthopsychiatry, 63,* 45–54.

Pihl, R. O., & Spiers, P. (1977). Some personality differences among the multidisciplinary team. *Journal of Clinical Psychology, 33,* 269–272.

Swezey, R. W., & Salas, E. (Eds.). *Teams: Their training and performance.* Norwood, NJ: Ablex.

Willoughby, R. H. (1978). The pediatric psychologist as "polyglot": Or training students to communicate clearly in a multidisciplinary world. *Journal of Clinical Child Psychology, 7,* 55–57.

I. Conflict Resolution and Problem-Solving

Goals

1. Describe the approaches to problem-solving, including the impact of each approach on community system relationships.
2. Understand the influences of personality, gender, and culture.
3. Recognize and discuss how one's personal style of communication will affect conflict resolution and problem-solving.

4. Suggest strategies for improving the effectiveness of personal communication and conflict resolution skills.

Special Interdisciplinary Conflict Issues in a Rural Setting

1. Colleague versus competitors
2. Isolation
3. Pressure of multiple roles
4. Need to involve in team planning other important providers who are involved in a particular case
5. Impact of large workload and lack of resources
6. Unrealistic expectations of team members
7. Differences in socioeconomic status of team members
8. Legal and regulatory accountability
9. Organizational/institutional policies and procedures
10. Willingness to share power
11. Federal regulations

Resources

Block, P. (1987). *The empowered manager: Positive political skills at work.* San Francisco: Jossey-Bass.

Bramson, R. M. (1981). *Coping with difficult people.* New York: Dell.

Fisher, R., & Ury, W. (1981). *Getting to yes: Negotiating agreement without giving in.* New York: Penguin.

McCormick, M. (1984). *What they don't teach you at Harvard Business School.* New York: Bantam.

Tannen, D. (1991). *You just don't understand: Women and men in conversation.* New York: Ballantine.

III

Prepracticum Lab

Goals

1. Obtain depth and training on methods as described below.
2. Conduct fieldwork to utilize these methods.
3. Understand and describe team functions and outcomes.

Prepracticum Lab and Advanced (see section IV) seminars are viewed as a continuum of training and education on methods to describe a rural community and its systems of care; an analysis of MH/SA service needs, strengths, and weaknesses; strategies to effect change, and team development and evaluation. The Prepracticum Lab is a series of exercises in which students apply knowledge, under supervision, to a rural community to accomplish the activities listed below, with models and case studies available for comparison.

A team of students is assigned a community to study and describe, including its ethnic and cultural factors and its systems of health, MH/SA, and social service. Methods of training focus on planning and collecting data to describe the community and on working as an interdisciplinary team. The first task is to plan a strategy to collect data, then to go out and collect data, making observations and interviewing key providers, agencies, and consumers. After this, students come back and describe their findings according to the following curriculum categories:

- Describing a rural community
- Describing community ethnic and cultural factors
- Describing community health, mental health, substance abuse, and social service systems

Following this activity, the students process their work from the interdisciplinary perspective using the following curriculum categories:

- Interdisciplinary activity and focus

  Format: Observe teams in action, form teams to experience the dynamics of team formation and operation, role-playing.

- Conflict resolution, with particular attention to federal regulations, JCAHO standards, and the use of forms

The Prepracticum Lab can run concurrently with section II, Preliminary Seminars.

Format: Case study, role-playing, apply conflict resolution strategies to any conflicts that arose in team-building exercise.

Resources

Flaskerud, J. H., & Kviz, F. J. (1984). Determining the need for mental health services in rural areas. *American Journal of Community Psychology, 12* (4), 497–510.

Nettekoven, L., & Sundberg, N. (1985). Community assessment methods in rural mental health promotion. *Journal of Rural Community Psychology, 6* (2), 21–43.

Rowley, B. D., & Baldwin, D. C. (1984). Assessing rural community resources for health care: The use of health services catchment area economic marketing studies. *Social Science Medicine, 6,* 525–529.

Waltman, G. H. (1986). Main street revisited: Social work practice in the rural setting. *Social Casework: The Journal of Contemporary Social Work, 67,* 466–474.

IV

Advanced Seminars

Goals

1. Provide integration of didactic and lab experience.
2. Identify strategy for collecting data on health problems.
3. Describe methods for conducting needs-assessments.
4. Conduct needs-assessment based on identification of physical and mental health problems and evaluation of current MH/SA service infrastructure.

Content

A. Assessment of rural community needs
B. Identification of rural community resources
C. Strategies to effect change in a manner sensitive to rural community values
D. Issues in professional development and survival
E. Development and functioning of interdisciplinary teams
F. Crisis intervention in a rural community

1. Articulate a working definition of crisis and crisis intervention. For some ideas, see:

Aguilera, D. C., & Messick, J. M. (1982). *Crisis intervention: Theory and methodology.* St. Louis, MO: Mosby.
Bradley, J., & Rotheram-Borus, M. J. (1990). Evaluation of imminent danger for suicide: A training manual. Tulsa, OK: National Resource Center for Youth Services.
Fisher, P. D., & Fisher, D. (1991, Sept./Oct.). EAP's and crisis management, *EAP Digest,* p. 42.

2. Describe how to implement a crisis intervention team in a rural community.

- Recognize the skills of all professionals and paraprofessionals across the community. This includes nurses, bachelor's level social services staff and school counselors, and masters' level practitioners.
- Develop an interagency initiative, including defining the scope of emergency (mental health, child protection, domestic violence, detox, etc). Identify lead agency for the first year. May rotate yearly. This agency is responsible for putting out schedule of on call and calling periodic meetings to review crisis intervention experiences and refine the system.
- Develop crisis intervention training of all providers.

- Identify the community resources, including 24-hour phone number. Examples include law enforcement dispatch and emergency rooms. Purchase technology appropriate to area (e.g., beeper) for workers to be notified of needs.
- Publish the existence of the 24-hour crisis service to the community.

3. Describe ways in which traditional crisis intervention techniques must be adapted to the cultural values and tradition of the community.

V

Practicum

This is the final portion of the curriculum, where students will work, under team supervision, in an interdisciplinary team model to address the MH/SA needs of a rural community, demonstrating and enhancing the knowledge and skills they have learned. See Attachment B for a description of a pilot practicum using the interdisciplinary curriculum.

Goal

1. Develop a supervised experience that will allow the student to demonstrate his or her knowledge and skills by producing a proposal for a project to address the specific needs of a rural site.

Resource

University of North Carolina. (1993). *Education for interdisciplinary rural health care: The role of the preceptor* (BHPr Contract No. 240-92-0030).

Additional Resources

Addleman, R. L., Tratnack, S. A., & Donat, D. C. (1991). Hospital-based multidisciplinary training in the care of the seriously mentally ill patients. *Hospital and Community Psychiatry, 42* (1), 60–61.

Alfred, U. (1988). Assessing mental health needs in the rural community: A critique of assessment approaches. *Issues in Mental Health Nursing, 9* (3), 299–315.

Arredondo, R., Wedding, R. L., Justice, C. L., & Fitz, J. (1987). Alcoholism in Mexican-Americans: Intervention and treatment. *Hospital and Community Psychiatry, 38* (2), 180–183.

Bachrach, L. L. (1977). Deinstitutionalization of mental health services in rural areas. *Hospital and Community Psychiatry, 28* (9), 669–672.

Bachrach, L. L. (1985). A sociological perspective. In L. R. Jones & R. R. Parlour (Eds.). *Psychiatric services for underserved rural populations* (pp. 5–26). New York: Brunner/Mazel.

Barry, B., & Davis, A. E. (1978). Community mental health ideology: A problematic model for rural areas. *American Journal of Orthopsychiatry, 48* (4), 673–679.

Beale, C. L. (1975). *The revival of population growth in nonmetropolitan America* (Economic Research Publication No. ERS-605). Washington, DC: US Department of Agriculture.

Beale, C. L. (1981). *Rural and small town population change, 1970–1980.* (Economics and Statistical Service Publication No. ESS-5). Washington, DC: US Department of Agriculture.

Beale, C. L., & Fuguitt, G. V. (1986, June). Metropolitan and non-metropolitan population growth in the United States since 1980. In *New dimensions in rural policy: Building upon our heritage.* Studies prepared for the Subcommittee on Agriculture and Transportation of the Joint Economic Committee of the Congress of the United States.

Beeson, P. G. (1992). Rural mental health research: The next generation. *Outlook, 2* (3), 2–6.

Bender, L. D., Green, B. L., Hady, T. F., Kuehn, J. A., Nelson, J. K., Perkinson, L. B., & Ross, P. J. (1985, September). The diverse social and economic structure of nonmetropolitan America. (Rural Development Research Report No. 49). Washington, DC: Economic Research Service, USDA.

Bosak, J., & Pearlman, B. (1982). A review of the definition of rural. *Journal of Rural Community Psychology, 3* (1), 3–34.

Bridges, D. (1994). A public–academic partnership to train psychiatric residents in a rural mental health program. *Hospital and Community Psychiatry, 45* (1), 66–69.

Briones, D., Heller, P., Chalfant, H., Roberts, A., et al. (1990). Socioeconomic status, ethnicity, psychological distress, and readiness to utilize a mental health facility. *American Journal of Psychiatry, 147* (10), 1333–1340.

Bryan, P. E. (1989). Psychological assessment of Black Americans. *Psychotherapy in Private Practice, 7* (3), 141–154.

Bui, K. T., & Takeuchi, D. T. (1992). Ethnic minority adolescents and the use of community mental health care services. *American Journal of Community Psychology, 20* (4), 403–417.

Buxton, E. (1970). Delivering social services in rural areas. In L. Ginsberg (Ed.), *Social work in rural communities: A book of readings.* New York: Council on Social Work Education.

Carlton-LaNay, I. (1992). Elderly Black farm women: A population at risk. *Social Work, 37* (6), 517–523.

Carscaddon, D. M., George, M., & Wells, G. (1990). Rural community mental health consumer satisfaction and psychiatric symptoms. *Community Mental Health Journal, 26* (4), 309–318.

Cecil, H. F. (1988). Stress: Country style. *Journal of Rural Community Psychology, 9* (2), 51–60.

Cohen, P., & Hesselbart, C. (1993). Demographic factors in the use of children's mental health services. *American Journal of Public Health, 83*, 49–52.

Collins, T. F. (1981). The media and mental health education. *Journal of Rural Community Psychology, 2* (1), 42–45.

Copp, J. H. (1976). The diversity of rural society and health needs. In W.W. Hassinger & L. R. Whiting (Eds.), *Rural health services: Organizations, delivery and use.* Ames, IA: Iowa State University Press.

Cordes, S. M. (1990). Come on in the water's just fine. *Academic Medicine: Journal of the Association of American Medical Colleges, 65* (3), 51–59.

Cowan, S. C. (1979). The rural poor and mental health. *Human Services in the Rural Environment, 1* (2), 10–18.

Coward, R. T., DeWeaver, K. L., Schmidt, F. E., & Jackson, R. W. (1983). Distinctive features of rural environments: A frame of reference for mental health practice. *International Journal of Mental Health, 12* (1–2), 3–24.

Curtis, P. (1990). The consequences of acculturation to service delivery and research with Hispanic families. [Special Issue: Culture and clinical social work.] *Child and Adolescent Social Work Journal, 7* (2), 147–159.

DeLeon, P. H., Wakefield, M. K., Schultz, A. J., Williams, J., & Vandenbos, G. R. (1989). Rural America: Unique opportunities for health care delivery and health services research. *American Psychologist, 44* (10), 1298–1306.

DeLeon, P. H., Wakefield, M. K., & Vandenbos, G. R. (1993). Health care in rural America: A national priority. In S. J. Jones (Ed.), *Sociocultural and service issues in working with rural clients: A resource guide for human service professionals* (pp. 77–92). Albany, New York: State University of New York, Albany.

Dufrene, P. M., & Coleman, V. D. (1992). Counseling Native Americans: Guidelines for group process. [Special issue: Group counseling with multicultural populations.] *Journal for Specialists in Group Work, 17* (4), 229–234.

Farberow, N. L. (1985). Mental health aspects of disaster in smaller communities. *American Journal of Social Psychology, 4*, 43–55.

Fandetti, D., & Goldmeier, J. (1988). Social workers as culture mediators in health care settings. *Health and Social Work, 13* (3), 171–179.

Fitchen, J. M. (1981). *Poverty in rural America: A case study*. Boulder, CO: Westview.

Fitchen, J. M. (1986). When rural communities collapse: Implications for mental health. *Rural Community Health Newsletter, 13* (2), 5–9.

Fitchen, J. M. (1990). Poverty as a context for old age in rural America. *Journal of Community Psychology, 11* (1), 31–50.

Fitchen, J. M. (1991). *Endangered spaces, enduring places: Change, identity, and survival in rural America*. Boulder, CO: Westview.

Flaskerud, J. (1986). The effects of culture-compatible intervention on the utilization of mental health services by minority clients. *Community Mental Health Journal, 22* (2), 127–141.

Flax, J. W., Wagenfeld, M. O., Ivens, R. E., & Weiss, R. J. (1979). *Mental health and rural America: An overview and annotated bibliography*. (DHEW Publication No. ADM 78-753). Rockville, MD: National Institute of Mental Health.

Freed, A. (1992). Discussion: Minority elderly. *Journal of Geriatric Psychiatry, 25* (1), 105–111.

George, L. K., Hughes, D. C., & Blazer, D. G. (1986). Urban/rural differences in the prevalence of anxiety disorders. *The American Journal of Social Psychiatry, 6* (4), 249–258.

Gibbons, S., Wylie, M. L., Echterling, L., & French, J. (1986). Patterns of alcohol use among rural small town adolescents. *Adolescence, 21* (84), 889–899.

Goeppinger, J. & Baglioni, A. J. (1985). Community competence: A positive approach to needs assessment. *American Journal of Community Psychology, 13* (5), 507–523.

Gorelick, D. A. (1992). Sociodemographic factors in drug abuse treatment. *Journal of Health Care for the Poor and Underserved, 3* (1), 49–58.

Grobsmith, E. S., & Dam, J. (1990). The revolving door: Substance abuse treatment and criminal sanctions for Native American offenders. *Journal of Substance Abuse, 2* (4), 405–425.

Guilmet, G., & Whited, D. (1989). The people who give more: Health and mental health among the contemporary Puyallup Indian tribal community. *American Indian and Alaska Native Mental Health Research, 2* (2), 141.

Hargrove, D. S. (1986). Rural community psychology and the farm foreclosure crisis. [Special Issue: Prevention and promotion.] *Journal of Rural Community Psychology, 7* (2), 16–26.

Heath, S. B. (1989). Oral and literate traditions among Black Americans living in poverty. *American Psychologist, 2*, 367–373.

Heyman, S. R. (1986). Addressing preventive interventions in rural community psychology. [Special Issue: Prevention and Promotion.] *Journal of Rural Community Psychology, 7* (2), 7–15.

Heyman, S. R., & VandenBos, G. R. (1989). Developing local resources to enrich the practice of rural community psychology. *Hospital and Community Psychiatry, 40* (1), 21–23.

Howard, G. S. (1991). Culture tales: A narrative approach to thinking, cross-cultural psychology, and psychotherapy. *American Psychologist, 3*, 187–197.

Hsieh, H., Cheng, S., Sharma, A., Sanders, R., et al. (1989). The relation of rural alcoholism to farm economy. *Community Mental Health Journal, 25* (4), 341–347.

Jennings, F. L. (1992). Ethics of rural practice. [Special Issue: Psychological practice in small towns and rural areas.] *Psychotherapy in Private Practice, 10* (3), 85–104.

Johnson, B. (1987). Sexual abuse prevention: A rural interdisciplinary effort. *Child Welfare, 66*(2), 165–173.

Jordan, S., & Hargrove, D. (1987). Implications of an empirical application of categorical definitions of rural. *Journal of Rural Community Psychology, 8* (2), 14–29.

Kirchner, J. H. (1981). Procedures and utilization of needs assessment in a rural area. *Journal of Rural Community Psychology, 2* (1), 46–50.

Koverola, C. (1992). Counseling aboriginal people of North America. [Special Issue: Multicultural counseling.] *Journal of Psychology and Christianity, 11* (4), 345–357.

Kovess, V., & Lafleche, M. (1988). How do teams practice community psychiatry? *Canada's Mental Health, 26* (2–3), 9–16.

LaFromboise, T. D. (1988). American Indian mental health policy. *American Psychologist, 43* (5), 388–397.

Leventhal, R. (1986). Beating the odds in rural America. 27th Annual Meeting of the Group Without a Name International Psychiatric Research Society (1985), Toronto Canada. *Psychiatric Journal of the University of Ottawa, 11* (2), 68–72.

Lichenstein, E., Nettekoven, L., & Sundberg, N. (1986). Training mental health promotion in rural settings. [Special Issue: Prevention and promotion.] *Journal of Rural Community Psychology, 7* (2), 37–54.

Lopez, S., Grover, K., Holland, D., Johnson, M., et al. (1989). Development of culturally sensitive psychotherapists. *Professional Psychology Research and Practice, 20* (6), 369–376.

Lorenzo, G. (1989). Current issues in the assessment and treatment of ethnic minority populations. *Psychotherapy in Private Practice, 7* (3), 133–140.

Martinez-Brawley, E. E. (1986). Beyond cracker-barrel images: The rural social work specialty. *Social Casework, 67* (2), 101–107.

Minton, B. A., & Soule, S. (1990). Two Eskimo villages assess mental health strengths and needs. *American Indian and Alaska Native Mental Health Research, 4* (2), 7–24.

Munetz, M. R., Birnbaum, A., & Wyzik, P. F. (1993). An integrative ideology to guide community-based multidisciplinary care to severely mentally ill patients. *Hospital and Community Psychology, 44* (6), 551–555.

Murray, D., & Keller, P. (1991). Psychology and rural America: Current status and future directions. *American Psychologist, 46* (3), 220–231.

Nelson, S. H., McCoy, G. F., Stetter, M., & Vanderwagen, W. C. (1992). An overview of mental health services for American Indians and Alaska Natives in the 1990s. *Hospital and Community Psychiatry, 43* (3), 257–261.

Office of Ethnic Minority Affairs (1993). Guidelines for providers of psychological services to ethnic, linguistic, and culturally diverse populations. *American Psychologist, 48* (1), 45–48.

Orlandi, M. A., Weston, R., & Epstein, L. (Eds.). (1992). *Cultural competence for evaluators: A guide for alcohol and other drug abuse prevention practitioners working with ethnic/racial communities*. Rockvillle, MD: Office of Substance Abuse Prevention.

O'Sullivan, M., & Lasso, B. (1992). Community mental health services for Hispanics: A test of the culture compatibility hypothesis. *Hispanic Journal of Behavioral Sciences, 14* (4), 455–468.

Palacios, M., & Franco, J. (1986). Counseling Mexican-American women. *Journal of Multicultural Counseling and Development, 14* (3), 124–131.

Paulsen, J. (1988). A service response to a culture in crisis. *Journal of Rural Community Psychology, 9* (1), 16–22.

Pedersen, P. (1990). The multicultural perspective as a fourth force in counseling. *Journal of Mental Health Counseling, 12* (1), 93–95.

Perez, A., Carr, K. D., & Sorenson, J. L. (1993). Cultural issues in an outpatient program for stimulant abusers. *Journal of Psychoactive Drugs, 25* (1), 35–44.

Phillips, K. & Rosenblatt, A. (1992). Speaking in tongues: Integrating economics and psychology into health and mental health services outcomes research. *Medical Care Review, 49* (2), 191–231.

Pinkerton, R. S., Moorman, J. C., & Rockwell, W. J. (1987). Multidisciplinary training in the college mental health service. *Hospital and Community Psychiatry, 38* (6), 656–661.

Randolph, H. (1985). The Dannevirke study: Implications for rural mental health. *Community Mental Health in New Zealand, 1* (2), 15–31.

Reed, D. (1992). Adaptation: The key to community psychiatric practice in the rural setting. *Community Mental Health Journal, 28* (2), 141–150.

Rogler, L., Malgady, R., & Costantino, G. (1987). What do culturally sensitive mental health services mean? The case of Hispanics. *American Psychologist, 42* (6), 565–570.

Rounds, K. (1988). AIDS in rural areas: Challenges to providing care. *Social Work, 33* (3), 257–261.

Santos, A., Deci, P., Lachance, K., Dias, J., et al. (1993). Providing assertive community treatment for severely mentally ill patients in a rural area. *Hospital and Community Psychiatry, 44* (1), 34–39.

Sayger, T. V., & Heid, K. O. (1990). Counseling the improvished rural client: Issues for family therapists. *Psychotherapy Patient, 7* (1–2), 161–168.

Smith, K. E., & Dibacco, J. (1974). The multidisciplinary training team: Issues and problems. *Journal of School Psychology, 12* (2), 158–167.

Sullivan, M., Ware, M. L., Giustini, I., Lascelles, M., et al. Perceived impact of an outreach rehabilitation program: A step toward program evaluation. *Canadian Journal of Rehabilitation, 4* (2), 67–74.

Swanda, R. M., & Kahn, M. W. (1986). Differential perception of life crisis events by sex, diagnosis, and ethnicity in rural mental health clients. [Special Issue: Prevention and promotion.] *Journal of Rural Community Psychology, 7* (2), 63–68.

Thompson, E. A., & McCubbin, H. I. (1987). Farm families in crisis: An overview of resources. [Special issue: Rural families: Stability and change.] *Family Relations Journal of Applied Family and Child Studies, 36* (4), 461–467.

Trimble, J. E. (1990). Application of psychological knowledge for American Indians and Alaska natives. *Journal of Training and Practice in Professional Psychology, 4* (1), 45–63.

Wagenfeld, M. (1988). Mental health and crisis of rural America. *Journal of Rural Community Psychology, 9* (2), 5–12.

Wagenfeld, M. O. (1988). Rural mental health and community psychology in the post community mental health era: An overview and introduction to the special issue. *Journal of Rural Community Psychology, 9* (2), 5–13.

Wallace, B. C. (1993). Cross-cultural counseling with the chemically dependent: Preparing for service delivery within a culture of violence. *Journal of Psychoactive Drugs, 25* (1), 9–20.

Waltman, G. H. (1986). Main street revisited: Social work practice in rural areas. *Social Casework, 67* (8), 466–474.

Weinert, C., & Long, K. (1987). Understanding the health care needs of rural families: Stability and change. *Family Relations Journal of Applied Family and Child Studies, 36* (4), 450–455.

White-Means, S. (1991). The economic returns from investments in physical and mental health: A case study of migrant farm workers in rural New York. *Journal of Health and Social Policy, 2* (3), 39–51.

Winiarski, M. G. (1994). Integrating mental health services with HIV primary care: The Bronx experience. *AIDS Patient Care, 7* (6), 322–325.

Worthington, C. (1992). An examination of factors influencing the diagnosis and treatment of Black patients in the mental health system. *Archives of Psychiatric Nursing, 6* (3), 195–204.

Young, T. J. (1991). Native American drinking: A neglected subject of study and research. *Journal of Drug Education, 21* (1), 65–72.

Attachment A: Comparison of Mental Health Factors for Las Vegas, New Mexico; Jackson, Wyoming; and Lame Deer, Montana

I. Introduction

This report provides background information on major mental health issues for team training curricula needs and development at each site. There are three major aims in presenting this material.

One is to provide information on the mental health needs and problems of each site within the context of the *Healthy People 2000* objectives for mental health. With this the Project Planning/Advisory Task Force can decide which problems will be emphasized in the curriculum at each site based on these objectives. A portion of the curricula will emphasize the contents of the specific problems of each site. The *Healthy People 2000* topics covered by this report are: (a) suicide; (b) mental disorders among children, adolescents, and/or adults; (c) adverse health effects from stress; (d) depression; (e) child abuse and neglect; and (f) partner-abuse behavior.

The second aim of this report is to assist students and faculty of the team training projects by providing them with information on the types of problems at each location. This provides a background on the nature and frequency of mental health problems likely to be encountered at each site.

The final aim is to demonstrate the usefulness of site-specific research. The collection and management of mental health related information on an ongoing basis has several important purposes. The collection of site-specific data provides information necessary for long-term planning. This is achieved by defining the impact of an array of mental health problems on the resources available at each site. These data can further be used as teaching and research tools by students, faculty, and local providers.

II. Infrastructure and Services

Site 1. Lame Deer, Montana: Northern Cheyenne Reservation

Contact

Arthur McDonald, PhD, President
Dull Knife Memorial College

Lame Deer, MT 59043
(406) 477–6215

Mental health service infrastructure (team training resources)

1. Outpatient mental health services
    a. Outpatient health center on-site (run by the Indian Health Service)
    Staff: 5 primary care physicians
    2 MSW social workers
    nursing staff
    Indian health representatives
    b. Community mental health clinic starting as part of Dull Knife Community College Pipeline Program, staffed by 3rd & 4th year PhD clinical psychology students from University of North Dakota and supervised by PhD psychologist at Dull Knife.
    c. Local healers
2. Outpatient/inpatient hospital mental health referrals
    a. Eastern Montana Mental Health Center (General OP)—Forsyth, MT
    b. Rivendale Psychiatric Center (Children/Adolescent IP)—Billings, MT
    c. Recovery Center (CD issues)—Lame Deer, MT
3. School programs
    - dropout project
    - substance abuse services
4. Dull Knife Community College
    - Two-year college
    - Strong curriculum in substance abuse, domestic violence
    - Psychology training/internship (rural mental health specialization) within the clinical PhD program of the University of North Dakota (Director: Jeff Holm, PhD)
5. Strengths/weaknesses:
    - Rural Indian reservation site
    - Knowledgeable psychologist and social work trainers
    - Opportunity to influence Indian Health Service use of psychologists
    - No inpatient opportunities
    - Nursing trainers required

Site 2. Jackson, Wyoming: Teton County

Contact

Michael Enright, PhD, Psychologist
Medical Arts Building, 557 East Broadway
Jackson, WY 83001
(307) 733–7771

Mental health service infrastructure (team training resources)

1. Outpatient mental health services
   a. Teton County Mental Health Clinic (PhD- and MS-level psychologists, MSW social workers)
   b. Private mental health practitioners (7 PhD. and MS levels)
   c. Outpatient and emergency room services at St. John's Hospital
   d. Local (nonlicensed) practitioners
   e. Curran-Seeley Foundation outpatient alcohol recovery program
2. Inpatient services at St. John's Hospital (45-bed hospital and regional facility)
3. St. John's Nursing Home (60-bed long-term care unit on hospital campus)
4. School/residential care programs for children with mental health problems
   a. Region V Boces (C-V Ranch)—residential school for developmentally disabled children
   b. Van Vleck House—assists and works with emotionally troubled youth of Jackson, WY
   c. Red Top Meadows—residential treatment center for boys ages 10–18
5. Task Force on Family Violence and Sexual Assault
   - 24-hour crisis line, safe-house for victims of battering and/or sexual assault, support groups, community education
6. Strengths/weaknesses for team training:
   - Inpatient hospital setting: PhD-level psychologists have full staff privileges
   - Nursing home with frail elderly patients
   - Active private practice psychologists fully integrated into medical care system
   - Local mental health center fully integrated into medical care system
   - In need of nurse-level trainers

Site 3. Las Vegas, New Mexico: Mora and San Miguel Counties

Contacts

Thomas Sturm, PhD
Director of Clinical Services
Las Vegas Medical Center
Las Vegas, NM 87701-1388
(505) 454–2100

Danny Roper, MSW
Acting Director
San Miguel/Mora
Community Mental Health Center
Las Vegas, NM 87701
(505) 454–8004

Mental health service infrastructure (team training resources)

1. Outpatient mental health services
   a. San Miguel/Mora Mental Health Center—PhD- and MA-level psychologists and psychiatrists; master's-level social workers; and MS-level nurses, case managers, and therapists. Primary care medical

providers, including a dentist. Affiliated with Las Vegas Medical Center. Serves local area from Las Vegas office, with two satellite offices in Pecos and Mora.

   b. A few private practice services
   c. Rio Grande Substance Abuse Services
   d. Local healers (Curanderes)

2. Inpatient facilities
   a. Las Vegas Medical Center (LVMC)—New Mexico's only state-run adult mental health hospital. Patient base covers entire state. Employs PhD- and MS-level psychologists and psychiatrists, MS-level social workers, PhD-level pharmacist, primary care physicians, nurses, and behavioral specialists. The facility has a wide variety of programs to serve adult, adolescent, elderly, forensic, and outpatient populations. Provides medical and mental health care services to remote multicounty area. Inpatient care organized in multidisciplinary teams. Core team includes psychiatrist, psychologist, social worker, and nurse. Outpatient care is provided through the mental health center mainly to boarding home and independent living patients who were formerly inpatients. The hospital is currently a training site for several educational institutions, including Highlands University, which offers psychology, nursing, and social work); the University of New Mexico's psychiatric students and medical residents; and occupational therapy students from the surrounding regions.
   b. Northeast Regional Hospital—Seventy-bed community general hospital located in Las Vegas, serving acute medical care patients from the area. Refers most patients requiring mental health assessment or treatment—50% of which are suicide attempts—to Las Vegas Medical Center.
3. 24-hour crisis line at LVMC
4. Strengths/weaknesses:
   - Inpatient psychiatric hospital setting with psychologists who have full staff privileges, (except prescribing drugs)
   - Current team approach for inpatient treatment
   - Nursing home for the mentally ill (mostly elderly)
   - Active outpatient mental health center integrated with the inpatient psychiatric hospital
   - Local boarding home and independent living patients
   - Medical/mental health outreach programs

III. Identification of Current Mental Health Problems

To facilitate identification of mental health related needs, we will describe the entire population at each site. Next, we will categorize the current users of mental health services based on diagnoses of mental health disorders. This will provide an estimation of the point prevalence for current mental health diagnoses. Prevalence, rather than incidence, of mental health disorders is estimated because there may be no clear moment of onset, the disorder may be intermittent, and, with few exceptions, these disorders are generally nonlethal. Prevalence for mental health related problems is based on annual rates of service-use and population data for each site.

Overview of Population and Data

A. Sites and regions. Regional information for the three sites includes the following geographic areas: (a) Las Vegas, NM: Mora and San Miguel counties; (b) Lame Deer, MT: Northern Cheyenne Reservation; and (c) Jackson, WY: Teton County. The three areas were compared in terms of demographic variations, mental health related disorders, and mental health related deaths.

B. Data sources. Each site was analyzed using vital statistics and clinical data for mental health related illnesses and deaths. A list of data sources is provided. (See Appendix 1.)

C. Limitations of data. Since this study was based, in part, on current use rates, it did not attempt to provide conclusive reporting on the status of mental health problems. For instance, if a person had a diagnosis and is not currently using services, an underestimation of prevalence would result. On the other hand, an individual with several disorders may be counted more than once, leading to overestimation. Nevertheless, the material presented provides a portrayal of recently diagnosed mental health disorders and related deaths.

Population Data

The population data were obtained from the 1990 U.S. Census Bureau and the Indian Health Services of Billings, MT. The description of population statistics includes population size, age, race, sex, education, employment status, and income.

A. Morbidity. Prevalence of mental health disorders was based on diagnoses or service use from local facilities. Morbidity data was requested for the most recent year, generally the fiscal year of July 1991–June 1992. The data were derived using diagnostic related group (DRG) and ICD-9 codes to classify cases. Markers for mental health disorders included DRG codes for: (a) acute adjustment reaction; (b) depressive neuroses; (c) disorders of personality and impulse control; (d) organic disturbances and mental retardation; (e) psychoses; (f) childhood disorders; (g) alcohol and drug related diagnoses; and (h) other mental disorders. Additional data pertaining to other mental health use trends were presented when available.

B. Mortality. Mortality data from the last five years were requested from each site's state office of vital records and from the Indian Health Services. Included in mortality data were deaths due to suicide, injury and accidents, alcohol, homicide, and legal intervention.

IV. Site Analyses and Comparisons

This section identifies specific issues for the three target sites. Data describing the population, mental illness, and deaths were compared for each site. Descriptions and summary of data follow.

Morbidity Data

Site 1. Las Vegas, New Mexico: Mora and San Miguel counties

Adult Morbidity

DRG	*n*	Annual Rate/ 10,000
425) acute adjustment reaction	8	3.8
426) depressive neuroses	26	12.4
427) neuroses other than depressive	20	9.5
428) disorders of personality & impulse control	9	4.3
429) organic disturbances & mental retardation	26	12.4
430) psychoses	424	201.9
434–437) substance abuse	20	9.5
Other, e.g., no diagnosis, diagnosis deferred	159	75.8
	N = 692	329.6

Child/Adolescent Morbidity Data: Aged <19

DRG	*n*	Annual Rate/ 10,000
426) depressive neuroses	2	2.2
427) neuroses other than depressive	4	4.4
430) psychoses	4	4.4
431) childhood disorders	8	8.9
Other, e.g., no diagnosis, diagnosis deferred	61	67.7
	N = 79	87.6

Site 2. Lame Deer, Montana: Northern Cheyenne Reservation

Adult Morbidity Data: Primary Diagnoses—Unduplicated Count

DRG	*n*	Annual Rate/ 10,000
425) acute adjustment reaction	17	74.1
426) depressive neuroses	28	122.2
427) neuroses other than depressive	6	26.2
428) disorders of personality and impulse control	2	8.7
429) organic disturbances and mental retardation	2	8.7
430) psychoses		
432) other mental disorders, e.g., sleep, eating, or sexual	1	4.4
434–437) substance abuse	45	196.3
Adult battering	2	8.7
Injury nonspecified	5	21.8
V-codes	57	248.7
	N = 165	719.8

Child/Adolescent Morbidity Data: Aged <19

DRG	*n*	Annual Rate/ 10,000
431) childhood disorders	18	99.1
Child battering	5	27.5
Depression	7	18.4
Alcohol	1	2.6
Trauma	19	50.1
Teenage pregnancy	60	326.4
	N = 110	524.1

Site 3. Jackson, Wyoming: Teton County

Adult/Child/Adolescent Morbidity Data: State MIS Data for Teton County and St. John's Hospital–Nursing Home, Jackson, Wyoming

DRG	*n*	Annual Rate 10,000
425) acute adjustment reaction	48	57.1
426) depressive neuroses	20	23.8
427) neuroses except depressive	243	289.1
428) disorders of personality and impulse control	18	21.4
429) organic disturbances and mental retardation	3	3.6
430) psychoses	83	98.7
431) childhood disorders*		
432) other mental disorders, e.g., sleeping, eating, sexual	12	14.3
434–437) substance abuse	45	53.5
449–451) poison or suicide attempt	11	13.1
Other, e.g., V-codes, diagnosis deferred	104	123.7
	N = 587	698.3

*Although the records were not specific in indicating this age group, 4 cases of DRG 427, and 7 of DRG 428 may have been childhood disorders. Records indicate 58 individuals aged <19 whose diagnoses were unknown.

Child/Adolescent Morbidity Data: Aged <19—St. John's Hospital, Jackson, Wyoming

DRG	*n*	Annual Rate/ 10,000
425) acute adjustment reaction	4	14.5
426) depressive neuroses	3	10.8
427) neuroses except depressive	—	—
428) disorders of personality and impulse control	—	—
429) organic disturbances and mental retardation	—	—
430) psychoses	1	3.6
431) childhood disorders	—	—
432) other mental disorders, e.g., sleeping, eating, sexual	1	3.6
434–437) substance abuse	3	10.8
449–451) poison or suicide attempt	4	14.5
	N = 16	57.8

Mortality Data

Site 1. Las Vegas, New Mexico: Mora and San Miguel counties

Mortality Rates for 1987–1991 (5 years) by Age (*N* = 158)

	Age Group			*All Ages*	
Category	0–14	15–64	65+	Total Deaths	Annual Rate /10,000
Alcohol related	N/A	N/A	N/A		
Suicide	0	32	1	33	2.2
Injury & accident	5	70	29	104	6.9
Homicide & legal intervention	1	18	2	21	1.4

Site 2. Lame Deer, Montana: Northern Cheyenne Reservation

Mortality Rates for 1988–1990 (3 years; *N* = 84). Data for Crow and Northern Cheyenne*

Category	Total Deaths	Annual Rate/ 10,000
Alcohol related	22	5.8
Suicide	2	0.5
Injury & accident	52**	13.7
Homicide & legal intervention	8	2.1

* Data not available for Cheyenne only, or by age group. Cheyenne represent 28% of this population.
**One case was possibly homicide or suicide.

Site 3. Jackson, Wyoming: Teton County

Mortality Rates for 1987–1991 (5 years) by Age Group (*N* = 37)

	Age Groups			*All Ages*	
Category	0–14	15–64*	65+	Total Deaths	Annual Rate/ 10,000
Alcohol related	N/A	N/A	N/A		
Suicide	0	8	2	10	1.8
Injury & accident	2	17	4	23	4.1
Homicide & legal intervention	1	3	0	4	0.7

*Teton County 15–19-year olds had 2 suicides and 3 accidents. 15–24-year olds had 1 suicide and 2 accidents. Data were presented in this format due to changes in the age categories of vital records, and to provide comparable data for all three sites.

Analyses and Summary of Data

The three sites varied in the following aspects:

1. Demographic data

a. Population. Mora and San Miguel counties had the largest population of 30,007, with an urban area (Las Vegas city) of 14,753. This urban area exceeded the total population size for either of the other two sites. The next largest site was Teton County with 11,172, while the Northern Cheyenne Reservation had the smallest population of 4,108.

b. Age distribution. Mora and San Miguel counties had the greater proportion of persons over 65 years old (12%), while Teton County and the Northern Cheyenne Reservation had similar elderly populations (6% and 5%, respectively). In contrast, the Northern Cheyenne Reservation had the highest percentage of youths under age 18 (44%), while Mora and San Miguel Counties and Teton County were more similar, with 30% and 25% youths under 18, respectively.

c. Sex. Mora and San Miguel counties and the Northern Cheyenne Reservation had equal ratios of males to females, while Teton County had a ratio of 52 males to 48 females.

d. Race and origin. Mora and San Miguel counties had a high proportion of people with Hispanic origins (80–85%). The Northern Cheyenne Reservation is predominantly Native American (90%). Teton County is mostly comprised of Whites (98%).

e. Education. The Northern Cheyenne Reservation had the largest proportion (47%) of youths between the ages of 16 and 19 who were neither enrolled in high school nor high school graduates. Teton County had 14.4% of these "at risk" youths, and Mora and San Miguel counties had the lowest percentage of these youths (11.5% and 7.9%, respectively). In contrast, Teton County had the highest proportion of people over the age of 25 with at least 12 years of education (91.9%). Mora and San Miguel counties had smaller numbers in this group (59.7% and 68.4%, respectively). The Northern Cheyenne Reservation had the smallest proportion in this category (57%).

f. Employment. Mora and San Miguel counties had an unemployment rate of 16.7% and 12.1%, respectively. Teton County had only 2% unemployment. Data for the Northern Cheyenne Reservation indicated the highest rate of unemployment—71% for males and 49% for females.

g. Income. In Mora and San Miguel counties, 38.6% and 30.2% of the population had an income less than $10,000 per year. Teton County had a lower percentage (8.2%) earning less than $10,000 per year, and the Northern Cheyenne Reservation had the highest (63%).

Data were similar for those earning less than $5,000. Mora and San Miguel counties had a higher percentage (20.8% and 14.0%), while Teton had only 3%. Data were not available for the Northern Cheyenne Reservation.

2. Morbidity data

a. Adult

1. Acute adjustment reaction
   - Examples included under this DRG heading are delirium, panic and anxiety, stress reaction, and nervousness disorders.
   - Mora and San Miguel counties had the lowest rate of diagnoses (3.8/10,000). Teton County had the next lowest rate (57.1/10,000), and the Northern Cheyenne Reservation had the highest of 74.1/10,000).
2. Depressive neuroses
   - Included under this DRG heading are neurotic, chronic, prolonged, and brief depression.
   - Mora and San Miguel counties had the lowest prevalence (12.4/10,000); Teton County had the next lowest rate (23.8/10,000); and the Northern Cheyenne Reservation had the highest (122.2/10,000).
3. Neuroses, other than depressive
   - Included under this DRG heading are phobic, neurotic, psychogenic, obsessive/compulsive, and academic/work inhibition disorders.
   - Mora and San Miguel counties had the lowest rate (9.5/10,000); Teton County had the highest rate (289.1/10,000); and the Northern Cheyenne Reservation had an intermediate rate of 26.2/10,000.
4. Disorders of personality and impulse control
   - Included under this DRG heading are multiple, schizoid, introverted, explosive, and compulsive personalities. Also covered are anorexia and kleptomania impulse controls.
   - Mora and San Miguel Counties had the lowest rate (4.3/10,000); Teton County had the highest (21.4/10,000); and the Northern Cheyenne Reservation was intermediate (8.7/10,000).
5. Organic disturbances and mental retardation
   - Included under this DRG heading are senile and presenile dementia, delirium, delusion, and depression. Also included are organic syndromes, autism, and Down's syndrome.
   - Mora and San Miguel Counties had the highest rate (12.4/10,000); Teton County had the lowest (3.6/10,000); and the Northern Cheyenne Reservation was intermediate (8.7/10,000).
6. Psychoses
   - Included under this DRG heading are simple schizophrenia, hebephrenia, catatonia, paranoid schizophrenia, depressive psychoses, and manic and bipolar disorders.
   - Mora and San Miguel Counties had the highest rate (201.9/10,000); Teton County had the next highest (98.7/10,000), and the Northern Cheyenne Reservation had no cases.

7. Other mental disorders diagnoses
   - Included under this DRG heading are sleeping, eating, and sexual disorders.
   - Mora and San Miguel Counties reported no cases with this diagnosis. Teton County had the highest rate (14.3/10,000), and the Northern Cheyenne Reservation had the lowest rate (4.4/10,000).
8. Substance abuse
   - Included under this DRG heading are various drug and alcohol abuses, dependencies, and withdrawal symptoms.
   - Mora and San Miguel Counties had the lowest rate (9.5/10,000); Teton County was intermediate (53.5/10,000); and the Northern Cheyenne Reservation had the highest rate of 196.3/10,000.
9. Poison or suicide attempt
   - Teton County had the only reported case, with a rate of 13.1/10,000.
10. Adult battering
    - The Northern Cheyenne Reservation had the only reported cases with a rate of 8.7/10,000.
11. Injury, unspecified
    - The Northern Cheyenne Reservation had the only reported cases with a rate of 21.8/10,000.
12. Other, e.g., V-codes, no diagnosis, or diagnosis deferred
    - This group was not compared since the category included different subjects, depending on site.

b. Adult morbidity data summary. Overall Mora and San Miguel counties' most severe problem concerned those disorders under the DRG heading of psychoses (201.9/10,000). For Teton County the highest rate of diagnoses was for neuroses other than depressive (289.1/10,000). On the Northern Cheyenne Reservation the highest mental health disorder prevalence was for substance abuse (196.3/10,000).

c. Child/adolescent morbidity data. Included for those under the age of 19 were:

1. Acute adjustment reaction
2. Depressive neuroses
3. Neuroses except depressive
4. Psychoses

All the above had the same categorizations as adult diagnoses.

5. Childhood disorders

These included attention deficit, learning disorders, pica, pyromania, identity and social conduct disorder.

6. Child battering
7. Poison or suicide attempt
8. Other, e.g., V-codes, no diagnosis, and diagnosis deferred

The most frequent childhood diagnosis in Mora and San Miguel counties was for childhood disorders (8.9/10,000). Teton County's most frequent problems were acute adjustment reactions (14.5/10,000) and poison or suicide attempt (14.5/10,000). On the Northern Cheyenne Reservation, the most frequent diagnoses were for childhood disorders (99.1/10,000), trauma (50.1/10,000), and child battering (27.5/10,000).

3. Mortality data

- Alcohol related deaths were only available from the Northern Cheyenne Reservation. Their death rate was 5.8/10,000.
- Suicide was lowest on the Northern Cheyenne Reservation (0.5/10,000), intermediate in Teton County (1.8/10,000), and highest in Mora and San Miguel counties (2.2/10,000).
- Injuries and accidents were highest on the Northern Cheyenne Reservation (13.7/10,000), intermediate in Mora and San Miguel counties (6.9/10,000), and lowest in Teton County (4.1/10,000).
- Homicide and legal intervention was highest on the Northern Cheyenne Reservation (2.1/10,000), intermediate in Mora and San Miguel counties (1.4/10,000), and lowest in Teton County (0.7/10,000).

V. Proposed Curricula Topics

1. Lame Deer, Montana—Local curriculum for team training program
   a. Substance use and abuse on the reservation
   b. Foundations of the oral tradition
   c. Traditional Indian mental health practices
   d. Resource availability in rural frontier areas
   e. Working with primary care physicians in outpatient care settings
   f. Development and management of data for identification, research, and analyses of mental health issues
2. Jackson, Wyoming—Local curriculum for team training program
   a. Treatment of chronically mentally ill in rural setting
   b. Working with primary care physicians in a community acute care hospital setting
   c. Resource availability and access in rural frontier communities
   d. Development and management of data for identification, research, and analyses of mental health issues
3. Las Vegas, New Mexico—Local curriculum for team training program
   a. Team treatment of acute and long-term chronically mentally ill in a rural psychiatric institution
   b. Working with primary care physicians in an inpatient psychiatric setting
   c. Working with primary care physicians in rural outpatient settings
   d. Resource availability and access in rural frontier communities
   e. Development and management of data for identification, research, and analyses of mental health issues

Appendix A–1: Data Sources

Las Vegas, New Mexico: Mora and San Miguel Counties

Mortality data

Office of Vital Records and Health Statistics
New Mexico Department of Health
P.O. Box 26110
Santa Fe, NM 87502

Morbidity data

San Miguel–Mora Mental Health Services
1214 National Avenue
Las Vegas, NM 87701

Jackson, Wyoming: Teton County

Mortality data

Department of Health, State of Wyoming
Division of Health and Medical Services
Vital Records Services
2300 Capitol Avenue
Hathaway Building, 4th floor
Cheyenne, WY 82002-0480

Morbidity data

Fiscal Year 1992 MIS Data
Department of Health, State of Wyoming
Division of Behavioral Health
2300 Capitol Avenue
Hathaway Building, 4th floor
Cheyenne, WY 82002-0480

St. John's Hospital and Nursing Home
P.O. Box 428
625 East Broadway
Jackson, WY 83001

Population data for all sites were obtained from the 1990 U.S. Bureau of Census.

Lame Deer, Montana: Northern Cheyenne Reservation

Mortality data

Indian Health Services
P.O. Box 2143
Billings, MT 59103

Morbidity data

Lame Deer Health Center
P.O. Box 98
Lame Deer, MT 59043

Preliminary report

Pond, D. (1992). *Prevalence of adolescent alcohol abuse in the Lame Deer area/Northern Cheyenne Indian Reservation.* Unpublished report.

Attachment B: Pilot Practicum

by Jeff Startzel, PsyD

A pilot practicum, using the interdisciplinary curriculum, was conducted in Jackson, Wyoming during the summer of 1994 in order, in part, to assess the usefulness of the curriculum and to provide feedback to its developers. This is a description of what was done.

Selection of the Practicum Site

The project took place in Jackson, Wyoming from June through August 1994. Jackson was selected as the training site because it possesses a unique set of characteristics for evaluating the utility of the curriculum, such as a 48-bed medical/surgical hospital with psychological services available, a well-established community mental health center, and a number of social service agencies. In addition, an influx of tourists and the associated need for increased local labor resources during the summer months considerably expands the patient population in this area, thereby raising the incidence of mental health problems requiring intervention. Thus, while Jackson contains many features of a rural setting, the number of mental health problems occurring during the summer months is higher than would be found in most typical rural settings. Further, because of the number of potential training rotations available, an interdisciplinary collaborative model could be utilized with the mental health center and hospital designated as the central sites.

Selection of the Preceptees

The preceptees for the practicum were identified through a multidisciplinary graduate seminar in rural mental health offered at the University of Utah. This course was taught by three faculty members from the University of Utah in Salt Lake City, Utah: Bill Farley, PhD from the School of Social Work, Ted Packard, PhD, from the Department of Counseling Psychology, and Sandra Talley, APRN, MN from the College of Nursing. These faculty members also provided consultation and supervision for the practicum over the course of the summer. The three preceptees for the practicum were a master's-level psychology student pursuing a PhD in counseling psychology, an advanced practice psychiatric nursing student, and a bachelor's-level student who had just completed his first year toward a master's degree in social work.

Practicum Supervisors

The on-site training faculty included Jeff Startzel, PsyD, Sarah Stark, MSW, and Michael Enright, PhD, ABPP. Dr. Startzel, a licensed psychologist at Jackson Hole Community Counseling Center and Chief of Psychology Services at St. John's Hospital, served as the site director. Ms. Stark, a licensed social worker, served as the other primary supervisor and assisted in coordinating training activities. Dr. Enright was the on-site placement consultant and also coordinated the development of the practicum from the APA curriculum.

The social work and psychology students received weekly individual supervision from a licensed practitioner in their respective disciplines. There was not, however, an advanced practice psychiatric nurse available in the community to provide supervision. Hence, this student received on-site supervision from Dr. Startzel and was also supervised via phone by Ms. Talley at the University of Utah. The students also participated in weekly group supervision conducted by Dr. Startzel and Ms. Stark. Additional supervision was provided by other local psychologists, hospital social workers, and supervisors of other practicum rotations. Throughout the course of the practicum, supervision stressed an interdisciplinary, collaborative approach, both through didactic presentation and by encouraging the students to adopt a team method in diagnostics and treatment.

A variety of mental health professionals, including psychologists, social workers, and psychiatrists, as well as professionals from outside the community, presented relevant topical workshops to the students. Workshops covered areas such as understanding the hospital culture, licensing and practice issues in rural areas, psychopharmacology and psychotropic medications, the *DSM-IV*, assessment and intervention with the suicidal client, interagency linkage and collaboration in rural settings, and medical causes of psychiatric symptoms.

Practicum Rotations

The community resources that served as the primary training sites were the Jackson Hole Community Counseling Center and St. John's Hospital. Jackson Hole Community Counseling Center is a nonprofit community mental health center that provides a broad spectrum of psychological services, including psychotherapy, assessment, community outreach, and consultation. St. John's Hospital is a 48-bed medical/surgical hospital with no identified psychiatric unit, although there are rooms designated for psychiatric patients and psychological services are well integrated into the services provided by the hospital. Participating psychologists are members of the hospital medical staff and provide consultation and treatment appropriate to their scope of practice. Students may also provide services at the hospital as preceptee staff under appropriate supervision.

Outpatient Rotation

Each of the practicum students carried a small outpatient therapy caseload at the Counseling Center, treating from three to five clients per week. Other duties at this location included intake assessments, participating with a clinician in responding to crisis situations, assessment and diagnostics, community outreach, and other experiences as deemed appropriate. In addition, the students participated in staff meetings and group supervision with other clinicians. As part of all of these experiences, the students were encouraged to examine and integrate clinical care across their disciplines, sharing respective treatment models with the objective of making contributions from their disciplines toward a common goal. The students also had the opportunity to examine mental health issues as they interface with the legal system by taking part in forensic assessments and involuntary commitment proceedings.

Inpatient Rotation

Each student was granted the appropriate degree of privileges to work in the hospital under direct supervision. As a master's-level practitioner, the psychology student was given medical staff appointment and designated as psychology support personnel. In this setting, the students were exposed to a host of diagnostic issues and patient problems, including schizophrenia, mood and anxiety disorders, suicidal patients, and substance abuse. Frequently, the students jointly conducted patient evaluations, synthesizing data and treatment formulations. Throughout the period in which each patient was hospitalized, the students met daily as a team with their direct supervisors, nurses, and the attending physicians when they were available. During these meetings, collaborative decision-making was emphasized, with the students sharing information and determining their respective roles in providing treatment. In most instances, the students had the opportunity to follow the patient after discharge from the hospital. This role was viewed as a particularly important element of their training, with considerable emphasis placed on the manner in which interdisciplinary collaboration could enhance continuity of care following inpatient treatment and its impact on long-term care concerns. The students were also issued electronic pagers so that they could respond with the on-call psychologist to psychiatric emergencies at the hospital emergency room.

Other Rotations

In order to provide broad exposure to the range of mental health issues encountered in rural communities, several other placements were developed. Each student spent approximately three hours per week at the local nursing home. In this capacity, they jointly facilitated groups, conducted mental status exams, and participated in the development of treatment plans. To provide exposure to child and adolescent populations, each student also served a rotation at two residential treatment centers for children and adolescents, where they cofacilitated groups, participated in treatment meetings, and collaborated with each other in assisting the primary providers in treatment implementation. Other resources in the community which were utilized included social services agencies, law enforcement, and public health. Although the students did not serve rotations at these sights, they frequently had the opportunity to interface with these entities and assist in the linkage of services.

In addition to the collaborative opportunities provided through the practicum, each student participated in individual training experiences relevant to their respective professions. The psychiatric nursing student worked closely with a consulting psychiatrist in order to gain familiarity with issues related to prescription privileges. The social work student spent one day per week working at the hospital with other social workers and also worked with the local Department of Family Services. The psychology student conducted several psychological assessments. He also observed forensic assessments and involuntary commitment proceedings. The students were encouraged to share these experiences with each other in an effort to increase understanding of their professional identities and to stimulate their thinking about collaborative issues.

Utilization of the Model Curriculum

The intent of this field practicum was to evaluate the functional utility of the interdisciplinary team training curriculum. Although it would have been valuable to have the students conduct a community needs assessment as outlined in the curriculum, the time limitations of the practicum made such an assessment infeasible. The students were, however, encouraged throughout their placement to informally assess the mental health needs of the community and to develop an understanding of the present service delivery system. This process was viewed as particularly critical to the issue of rural practice. In this respect, the students had multiple opportunities to appreciate the need for creativity and interagency collaboration where services and resources are more limited than in urban areas, and at times, nonexistent. The most salient feature of the practicum that extended from the curriculum was related to the development of the interdisciplinary team. As discussed above, most of the training experiences stressed a collaborative model, requiring the students to address such issues as historical barriers to collaboration, group progress, design of team structure, specialization, more time required by increased communications across disciplines, and communication problems among team members. However, as the practicum progressed and team cooperation and coordination improved, the students became quite effective in confronting these issues. Overall, the students began the practicum with a solid academic understanding of the curriculum; the field placement provided them with multiple opportunities to put the issues identified in the curriculum into practice.

Practicum Evaluation

One of the early difficulties encountered in developing this placement was gaining the cooperation and support of the many professionals in the community whose involvement in the project was viewed as critical, such as the hospital staff, as well as the administrators and supervisors of the rotation sites. Some of these individuals expressed concerns that working with and supervising the students would add an additional burden to their program operations. The students, however, quickly came to be viewed as assets, enhancing the delivery of services. In part, this outcome was related to the student's willingness and ability to assume active roles at these rotation sites. With this in mind, their degree of academic preparation and participation in the rural mental health seminar appeared to be important elements in their ability to rapidly adjust to the demands of the practicum rotations. Overall, despite some initial trepidation, the students were well—and in many cases, eagerly—received by the various individuals, agencies, and service providers in the community, a factor that greatly contributed to the success of the project.

Another potentially problematic issue was the unavailability of an on-site advanced practice psychiatric nurse to provide direct supervision. However, this concern was effectively addressed by utilizing the psychologist and psychiatrist on-site for supervision and then providing an advanced practice psychiatric nurse (Ms. Talley) for weekly phone supervision.

Future practicums will also need to consider the length of the placement. The 10-week period in which the practicum took place, which was determined on the basis of the students' availability during the summer recess, seemed too brief to allow them to fully appreciate some of the problems that might develop in working within a collaborative model, such as professional boundary issues and difficulties in the group process. In addition, the time limitation prohibited the students from becoming as comfortable as they might have with their workload, with the community and its resources, and with implementing their newly acquired skills and knowledge. Finally, logistical issues, such as housing, stipends, and moving, must be addressed well in advance so that the students can immediately begin to focus their energies on the demands of the placement.

Overall, the pilot project was successful for a number of reasons. The students unanimously expressed a high degree of satisfaction with their experiences and stated that the practicum far exceeded their expectations in terms of breadth of experiences, opportunities to put into practice newly acquired skills and knowledge, exposure to rural mental health issues, and the multiple opportunities for team collaboration. All three students, when questioned, stated that they would readily consider the potential of rural practice and, indeed, viewed it as more desirable in many respects than urban practice. Responses from supervisors and others associated with the program have highlighted the advantages of such program elements as interdisciplinary case conferences and collaborating with other professionals. In summary, this pilot project appears to have been a worthwhile and successful extension of the model curriculum, suggesting that continuation and expansion of this practicum represents a viable and effective means for training mental health professionals in a collaborative approach to mental health care in rural areas.

Issues for Future Field Practicums

As previously noted, the degree of academic preparation and practicum experience of the students was critical to the success of the project. Due to the breadth of experiences and issues encountered during the practicum, it was essential that the students be mature, as well as relatively knowledgeable and comfortable with mental health issues. Therefore, the selection process for such placements should carefully consider the degree of preparation the students have had in the fundamentals of their respective disciplines, ability to adapt to a variety of novel experiences and situations, interpersonal skills, and interest in utilizing a team approach to rural mental health service delivery.

Two elements limited the ability of this practicum to answer several important questions regarding the utility of employing an interdisciplinary model in rural mental health delivery: funding and time. Questions that could be answered through a more formally funded research project include (a) Do practicums of this type increase the likelihood that students will choose rural practice, (b) does interdisciplinary collaboration enhance service delivery and quality of care, (c) is such a model viable for rural communities, (d) what barriers exist to discourage collaborative models, and (e) can this type of practicum help to break down historical barriers between professional groups? Given the inherent difficulties in effectively extending mental health services to rural populations and the increasing importance of this issue, continuing to develop and evaluate practicums of this type should be given priority.